IN LESS THAN ONE MONTH YOU CAN TRANSFORM YOUR LIFE!

Share the secrets of food, nutrition, exercise, relaxation, and stress management that have helped thousands at Janet Greeson's "A Place For Us" to build a positive self-image and empower their lives. Her 28-day medical plan can do the same for you with:

- The "A Place For Us" food plan, tailored to your special needs
- Exercises to help you find the "Real Me" in you
- Self-tests to increase self-awareness
- Vitamin and mineral therapies to reduce stress and cravings
- Movement therapies to develop a positive body image
- Meditation, visualization and other relaxation techniques
- Case histories of food addicts who are in recovery—to offer hope and help along the way

Reshape your attitudes as well as your body—with *IT'S NOT WHAT YOU'RE EATING, IT'S WHAT'S EATING YOU!*

JANET GREESON, holds a Ph.D. in Psychology from Columbia Pacific University. She is the originator and clinical director of Janet Greeson's "A Place For Us," with centers in Daytona Beach, Orlando and Los Angeles. She is a recovering food addict who has maintained a 150-pound weight loss for over 15 years.

IT'S NOT WHAT YOU'RE EATING, IT'S WHAT'S EATING YOU

The 28-Day Plan to Heal Hidden Food Addiction

Janet Greeson, Ph.D.

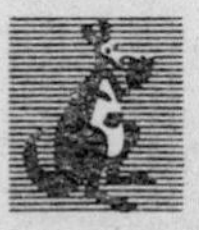

POCKET BOOKS
New York London Toronto Sydney Tokyo Singapore

An *Original* Publication of POCKET BOOKS

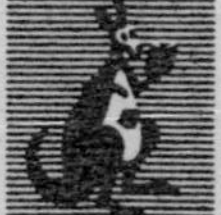

POCKET BOOKS, a division of Simon & Schuster Inc.
1230 Avenue of the Americas, New York, NY 10020

ISBN: 0-671-68224-5

First Pocket Books printing April 1990

15 14 13 12 11 10 9 8

Printed in the U.S.A.

Acknowledgments

This book was made possible first by the love of God and St. Theresa The Little Flower. Then the gentle love of my children, Gene, Jimmy and Roe, and especially my mother Rosemary, whose love has energized me my entire life.

I definitely could not have written this book without the generous support of writers Catherine Revland and Shannon Rothenberger. Their belief in me and hanging in there throughout this book was above and beyond. They are little flowers themselves and were the catalyst for numerous contributions. God really worked through them both. My agent, Frank Weimann, with his chaotic, wonderful energy was a great support and thanks to Hollywood Henderson for introducing us.

I will be forever grateful for the nourishment of family and friends who encouraged me and inspired me throughout. Special love to Terry Lamond, Father Leo Booth, Fred Earle, Ph.D., Kitty Duffy, Peggy Favata, Deneice Howard, Jerry Smith, Marty Van Henrik, Blanche Stokley, the "A Place For Us" staff, and past husbands who have helped me.

This is dedicated to food addicts and all the past patients of Janet Greeson's "A Place For Us."

Contents

Preface

Those of us who suffer from food addiction live in the prison of our own bodies. If you dislike or struggle with your body, you are in one, too. The prison is entrapping you in the false image you have of your body, an image no one else in the world sees but you. The tragedy of being in this prison is that the incarceration is not mandatory. You are in a state of self-imposed solitary confinement. You arrested yourself, you were the prosecuting attorney, the judge, the jury, and you are now the prison guard.

You built your prison with the tools of your own imagination, not to incarcerate but to protect yourself. Your building blocks were painful memories and negative messages you picked up from other people and from society at large. You compared yourself to others, and to the impossible standards given to you by the media, and found yourself lacking. Although everyone has flaws, you saw yours alone.

You fortify those walls every day with new messages of negativity, not just from others but from yourself, and your own criticism is the harshest of all. You reject messages of acceptance and love because they do not fit into the structure you have built for yourself.

Is it any wonder that people who suffer from food addiction are deeply depressed? In fact, unhappiness is the universal symptom expressed by people who come to my treatment centers. But through my experiences I have come to realize that depression is not a symptom of food addiction, but rather at the root of the problem. I used to weigh 350 pounds, and I always felt that my body was all anyone could see. This negative image was reinforced by people around me; whenever I went to the doctor, whether I had the flu, asthma, or a broken leg, it seemed like the physician would always wind up discussing my weight. It was only years later that I discovered that a combination of fear, anger and depression was my real problem. I was using the food to kill myself in a slow, numb way.

The stories within these pages are not about food but about broken hearts, broken dreams, how life becomes a struggle, and people who, no matter what they try to do, feel stuck in their mental prison. You can't treat food addiction by focusing on the food; that's like applying a band-aid to a deep, festering wound. And every new diet is just a different bandage; they might work for a while, or at least mask the wound, but the most beautiful band-aid in the world is not going to heal it.

The body heals itself from the inside out, never the other way around. The only way to treat a deep wound is to go to the root of it, painful as that may be, clean it out and apply a nurturing dressing. Given the right attention, the body miraculously heals itself, and when the bandages are removed there may be no sign at all of the damage that was there. No scars.

The wounded mind heals in a similar way. Broken dreams can be mended once the damage that has been done is cleaned out at its deepest source. Even the wounds of childhood can be healed. My mission is to make a difference in your life by helping you mend your dreams, from the inside out, so you can walk about freely, bouncing with life.

Deeply wounded people are desperate; they are willing to try almost anything to relieve their pain. They go on every new diet that comes along, or try intense exercise programs, but still no healing takes place. Diet and exercise are important, but they only treat the symptom. Even therapy alone does not work; when the mind alone is treated, people can stay imprisoned in their thoughts forever, intellectualizing but never experiencing what they feel. In treating thousands of patients I have come to believe that no one approach will work. The mind and body must work together. The mind is capable of telling us incredible lies, convincing us that merely thinking about something is experiencing it. For instance, people can talk about their anger and never really feel it; but when mind and body work together, a catharsis takes place. By simultaneously expressing anger (feeling) with action (body movement) as well as words (mind) you can truly experience anger, often for the first time, as well as experience the relief that comes when a strong and sometimes terrifying emotion is discharged. This book is designed to get the mind and body working together; the exercises at the end of each chapter will help you to experience life.

Many readers have told me they use this book not just with a buddy, as I recommend, but in discussion with friends they have come to trust in ways that enhance their relationships. Although it is possible to derive much benefit from working with a buddy alone, I enthusiastically support taking advantage of a group effort, if it is available. After many years of treating people with depression, I now have statistical data confirming my belief that no single approach to treatment will ever be as powerful as a group effort. It's amazing how the combined energy of a group can bring everyone in the group to a higher level of mind. But remember this: whether you choose to work with a buddy or a group, recovery takes action, and without it people are likely to remain prisoners of their own thoughts forever.

I have come into your life to help you plot your escape from the prison you may be in. You don't need a saw or a crowbar, for you are in possession of the key that will unlock the prison door. Healing begins with love, not from without but from within. Love of self will unlock the prison door. It may not open easily after being shut for so long, but your imagination, which put you where you are, can also set you free.

The sun is shining outside the prison walls, and the breezes are gently blowing. What are you waiting for? Let's go!

I

It's Not What You're Eating

1

I Am Not My Body

Please allow me to make an assumption about you. You are reading this book because you are unhappy over your relationship with food. What was once a source of enjoyment now gives you pain. Intrigued by the title, you have begun reading to look for the answer you have never found in the many diet books you have read: mainly, why you can't eat like "normal" people. You have picked it up because sooner or later (mostly sooner) your willpower fails and food controls your thoughts, your actions, and even haunts your dreams. You have picked it up because you suspect that, yes, there definitely is something "eating you."

Before we begin, it's very important that you leave behind all the concepts about food and dieting you've read elsewhere. My approach is so different that before I begin to explain it, I feel the need to reorient you in a totally new direction.

It's Not What You're Eating

This is not a book about food; it's about feelings. It's not about the stuffing, it's about the stuffee. It's not about how much you eat or what you eat or don't eat, or how often you eat, but what happens to you when you do eat. Any weight-loss plan that does not uncouple feelings from food is bound to fail. This is a book for people who eat not to nourish their bodies but to make themselves *feel* better. It is the first book to treat the use of food as a mood-altering substance, as an addiction.

Food addiction is a disease of the human spirit and it can't be cured by a physical solution alone. Like putting a Band-Aid on a deep wound, underneath the cosmetic treatment is a problem that is hurting and festering. It needs to be cleaned out before it will heal, and that can be painful, but it's the only way healing will take place. Healing any deep wound is not a pleasant process, but it is nowhere nearly as painful as leaving it untreated.

Don't be frightened by the idea that you might have a disease. Broken down, the word reveals its simple meaning: dis-ease, or the absense of comfort. Acknowledging you have a disease permits dignity and the right to obtain medical attention for something that is *not your fault*. It banishes all ideas of guilt, lack of control, and even the word "diet," which beyond the first explanatory chapter you will not even find in this book.

Three Reasons Why Diets Don't Work

It's true you can lose weight on them, sometimes a lot. The problem is gaining all those pounds back again, plus a few extra, which is all but inevitable. I know someone who lost a hundred pounds in six months on the Dr. Atkins diet and gained them all back in six weeks! Very few dieters manage to sustain a weight loss, particularly a dramatic one.

You undoubtedly know diets don't work, but think the reason is your lack of willpower. That's like blaming diabetics for their inability to metabolize sugar. The reason diets don't work has nothing to do with self-restraint and everything to do with body chemistry and the way the mind functions.

First, the physical aspect: The body can handle only one extended fast in a lifetime. Sudden or prolonged deprivation of food lowers its metabolism rate, which is the amount of calories it requires to burn each day in order to function. In the millions of years the human being has existed, this metabolic adjustment served an important evolutionary purpose. During periods of famine, it assured the survival of those whose bodies were ingesting fewer calories.

Because of our heritage, crash diets are self-defeating. They trigger our genetic alarm system, decreasing the amount of calories we need to function and causing our bodies to store extra fat as a hedge against future deprivation, thus keeping us a prisoner of calorie-counting forever. Fortunately, all is not lost. Exercise and proper nutrition will eventually restore our metabolism rate somewhat, though it's debatable if we will ever get back to where we started. Obviously, the sensible thing is never to go on a crash fasting diet in the first place.

The second reason diets fail occurs in the mind. Have you ever noticed that as soon as you go on a diet, you start obsessing about food more than ever? The reason is simple: People move toward their most dominant thought, even if that thought is about not having something. Diets are all about deprivation. Even the word sets up a bad connotation: "die-et," or as a psychologist friend of mine defines it, "You die because you et." Go on a diet and you'll start dying for whatever it is you crave, because you can't have it. Suddenly, all your mental energy is expended on fulfillment of that one dominant thought. As a result, even while managing to resist putting the forbidden food into your mouth, you're still a prisoner of food in your mind. You might not be burning the calories, but your mind is burning with thoughts about what you're not eating. No wonder diets make people so depressed!

In this book, I will not talk about diets. I will talk about food plans. Instead of focusing on deprivation, we will focus on what we *can* eat, and I'm sure you will find there are a lot of foods you like that are included in the daily menus listed within.

The third reason diets don't work is they focus on control. Because people with eating disorders think in terms of controlling what they eat, they are often very rigid in their attitude. After all, addiction to food is much more difficult to live with than addiction to alcohol or other substances from which people can totally abstain. There's an Overeaters Anonymous saying: "You can put the plug in the jug and keep it there, but you've got to take the tiger out of the cage three times a day and feed it without getting hurt." Because eating is necessary to life, food addicts often believe they must control the urge to eat to excess every time they put food in their mouths, but sooner or later that negativity will do them in and they'll attack food with a vengeance.

Inadvertently we've all had what we consider *bad* foods. Notice how we put moral labels on food. We give it such power. I tell myself, just because I made a mistake doesn't mean I *am* a mistake. In dealing with food, we're all going to make mistakes. The problem with most dieting is, people think because the diet is a failure, they're a failure. As hard as they try, and as motivated as they are, they just don't know how to exercise control over food.

There is a widespread myth about food addicts that control is their main issue. I disagree. Control is a symptom. The core issue is powerlessness. The food addict gives away the power to the food. Think of the power people give to that "just one" potato chip that will lead to a binge.

I don't believe in focusing on control. It makes as much sense as treating an allergic rash with a skin cream. You don't treat the symptom, you treat the addiction, and the addiction is about powerlessness. Instead of encouraging you to increase your willpower, I will encourage you to embrace your powerlessness. In order to conquer food addiction you do not conquer it: **"What you resist persists."*** Going into battle with food gives it power, be-

---

*Unattributed quotes that appear in boldface in this book are 12-step axioms, which, like the program, are anonymous.

cause it becomes a moral issue. That's why it's a mistake to label food good or bad; if people eat "bad" food, they tend to think they become bad themselves. As a consequence they may do penance, and sometimes the punishment they mete out is eating more, or doing without, which puts them back in the deprivation mode again.

We live in a society of learned helplessness. All our lives people tell us we can't do things, and we grow up giving away our power by learning to rely on someone else or society to have all the answers. My goal in this book is to encourage you to claim your own power. This may seem impossible at this point, but believe me, it will work for you as it has for me and many thousands of others.

Fifteen years ago I weighed 340 pounds and had been dieting half my life, losing the same 100 pounds over and over again. I was not so much living as existing, and knew I was eating myself to death. I lost the weight I needed to lose and kept it off—permanently—not by dieting. I have a food plan called 301—three meals a day, nothing in between, and one day at a time—and I follow a program that requires me to make major changes not so much in my eating habits as in my attitudes and my behavior. Although I will remain a food addict until the day I die, I am no longer a prisoner of my body, and that has liberated my mind from obsession and allowed me to create a full, rich, and happy life for myself. You can, too.

Food As an Addiction

You are probably still uncomfortable with the term "food addict." When I use the word "addiction," I mean the continued use of a mood-altering substance in spite of the negative consequences, coupled with a greatly diminished capacity to exercise free will over its use. Addiction is characterized by overdoing, in spite of lost health, jobs, relationships, and status. If there are no negative consequences to your behavior in relation to food, and if there is no disparity between your need to control your intake of food and your ability to do so, then you aren't an addict. If there is, I hope you will keep an open mind and consider the fact that you might be.

Another helpful definition of addiction comes from the *Big Book of Alcoholics Anonymous:* "a mental obsession coupled with a physical compulsion." Food addicts are constantly thinking about food and cannot stop eating once they start. That's the double whammy of the addiction; not only do your thoughts propel you to eat, physical changes take place when you eat that cause you to keep eating without the ability to stop when you're no longer hungry. An alcoholic can never understand how a person can sit and nurse one drink all night. A food addict can never understand how a person can cut a sliver out of a cake and not wind up eating the whole thing. And when that cake is gone, the food addict experiences no satisfaction, only disgust and shame. I relate that feeling to a cat's making love to a skunk: I didn't have all I wanted, but I had about all I could stand.

Because it is the earliest addiction, food is very often the primary one. Many alcoholics manage to stop drinking only to be confronted with their addiction to food in their recovery. It is also the most common addiction. More people die from it each year than all the other addictions combined, yet there's rarely an emphasis put on food as a potentially lethal substance. There are no labels on bakery trucks or photos of seven-layer cakes in magazines that announce, "Warning: Consumption may be dangerous to your health." Nor is there much social stigma attached to food addiction. Eating too much is generally considered a joke, but I didn't laugh at the sign I recently saw on the wall of a New York restaurant: "*Morte de Pasta*—proudly killing you since 1985."

Genetic Addiction

Food addiction runs in families. Women tend to abuse food more than men, who tend to turn to alcohol instead. Mothers who abuse food pass on their addiction to their children. If one or both of your parents were food addicts, the chances are great that you're one, too. A significant amount of medical research has been conducted on the theory that certain people are born addicted, so that by rights a biopsy could be done at birth to determine whether a person was going to grow up to be an addict. Not every addict is genetically addicted, but those of us who are have fewer of the chemical brain messengers known as endorphins, and that deficiency causes us to feel as if we're always "running on low." Certain mood-altering substances such as sugar, alcohol, opiates, and other drugs penetrate the blood barrier of the brain, causing a feeling of euphoria, which is intensified in the genetically addicted, for they are accustomed to feeling "low."

The molecular structures of sugar and alcohol are similar when they are broken down in the body. Because of their special neurochemical sensitivity, addicts develop an allergy to sugar that triggers a vicious cycle of craving: at first, eating sweets does make them feel better by raising their blood sugar, but when it drops again, the body cries out for more, repeating the cycle. Stress also triggers a sugar craving, causing mind-altering chemicals such as calecholine to stimulate the appetite. People eat a sweet snack to relieve the stress, and after the sugar drop-off they're back in the cycle of craving again. Heavy carbohydrate meals can also lead to sugar consumption. They trigger release of the chemical brain-messenger serotonin, an endorphin that reduces mental alertness. Then, when people get drowsy, they turn to sugar again for a quick pick-me-up. Because of its prevalence in society, and its connection to the joys of childhood, sugar is rarely seen as the drug it really is.

Some people are born endorphin deficient. From the very first time they ingest substances that raise their abnormally low endorphin levels, they feel a tremendous sense of well-being. With the continued use of a substance the addiction cycle has begun. Food addicts can vividly recall the special foods of their childhood, alcoholics that first drink and you'd be amazed at the intensity of the memory.

Increased Tolerance

Unfortunately, you never have enough of what you don't want, because the substance is not what you really want—it's the feeling. In addition, that initial euphoria cannot be sustained, for addiction is a progressive disease. As time goes on, it takes more and more food to sustain an increasingly diminishing intensity level of feeling good. Eventually that wonderful feeling of well-being that makes the early stages of addiction so seductive becomes a source of disenchantment, for it is never reached again, no matter how much of the mood-altering substance is taken. The first time an alcoholic drinks, he might get a buzz after two drinks. Later it will take six or seven to get comparatively high. In advanced stages he might drink the whole bottle and feel nothing at all.

The same increased tolerance takes place in food addicts. In the early stages, a few slices of cake will produce the good feelings they seek, then half the cake, and pretty soon, the whole thing. In advanced stages not even that gives them the intensity of feeling they crave. No matter what or how much they eat, they get no relief. Everyone has abused food at some time in their life, but when people have to eat more and more to elevate their mood, or as the disease progresses, to achieve a soporific numbness, you're looking at addiction. With today's increased awareness and education about fitness and nutrition, if overeating were just a bad habit, we would be making terrific strides, but we're not. The United States has the largest population of overeaters in the world. Even our children's percentage of body fat has increased.

The same pattern of increased tolerance is true for anorexics. They eat less and less, looking for the intensity. Bulimics often complain that they feel numb, saying the only time they feel intensely is when they vomit. It gets them high, but after a while even that violent experience leaves them feeling numb.

Withdrawal

Another sign of addiction is the state of discomfort a person experiences in the absence of the substance of choice. Nicotine addicts who light up a cigarette first thing in the morning are in a state of withdrawal, having not ingested their drug since the night before, and they need it just to start their day. Sugar withdrawal, which people experience when they go on a diet, produces headaches, listlessness, and irritability as intense as other kinds of drug detoxification. It's one of the reasons why going on a diet is such a miserable experience. People who are ravenously hungry right before bed, three or four hours after a big dinner, or who get up in the middle of the night to raid the refrigerator, are also going through withdrawal. The intensity of their need has nothing to do with actual hunger. If true hunger were being experienced, that intensity would be appropriate after a night's sleep, or a busy morning of work. Looking for the times during the day when you are experiencing the greatest desire for food is a good measure of whether that desire is out of real need or whether you're experiencing withdrawal.

Isolation

In the words of Robert Morley, "No man is lonely while eating spaghetti." That perfectly describes the relationship addicts have with their substance of choice. Addicts are emotional loners. Their feelings are attached to food, booze, drugs, work, other people, gambling, or whatever their obsessive-compulsive behavior uses as a distraction from their inner emptiness. Their energy is inner directed only with the substance and outer directed only with the need for others to tell them how they should look, feel, or think. Inside, there is a void where their own spirit should be. All their relationships are distorted. The food, the alcohol, the drugs, are always in between them and the relationship.

Addiction is a disease of isolation. Instead of having relationships with other people, the food addict withdraws from social contact to have a relationship with food. It isn't necessary to be alone to experience isolation. In fact, loneliness can be the most intense when one is surrounded by other people, none of whom the addict can feel close to. Intimacy is not possible when the people who desire closeness are not in touch with who they really are. In fact, they feel uncomfortable when they try to get close to others, and even when others think they are achieving intimacy, the addict knows it's not the real thing. Out of touch with their own authenticity, they feel like imposters. Frustrated in their attempts to seek intimacy with people, they try to have a love affair with food. The food calls to them. It has warmth. It is capable of nurturing. It lives! The problem of having a love affair with food is that it never satisfies. No amount will ever fill the emptiness.

It's What's Eating You

Food addicts are eating a whole lot more than food. They're eating feelings associated with food. If they're angry, they'll go for a crunchy food. If they're in need of mothering, they'll go for something soft, sweet, and milky. There's a well-known laboratory experiment that illustrates this linkage of food and feelings. A mother monkey died and her babies were dying because they would not take milk from a bottle. The scientists made a wire-mesh monkey and covered it with fur, then fed the baby monkeys through the wire mesh so they could get warmth and nurturing along with their food. All the babies flourished. Food addicts are like those baby monkeys. The connection between food and comfort is so deep they can't make the distinction. They go for food instead of going after what they really want, which is intimacy with people.

Food addicts will often develop cravings around food associated with early nurturing. For me it was mashed potatoes. My father loved them and we had them every day. As a grown woman, when I craved them, they weren't just mashed potatoes; they stood for love, nurturing, and security. Addicts have trouble sorting out the source of these feelings, particularly pleasurable ones that they find hard to accept and have to distort. Deep down, they really don't believe they deserve to feel good. When they do, they worry they're not going to get enough of those good feelings, or they come into contact with how needy they are, and that neediness scares them. Because their lives are so full of stress and crisis, when they do feel pleasure, they don't know how to relax and enjoy it without feeling guilty.

Food addicts will readily tell you what they think, but they have a hard time telling you what they feel. After so many years of denying their emotions, the only way they can feel is through the eating, denial, or purging of food. A binge is really an explosion of emotion. As soon as bingers grasp that concept, they can use identification of feelings as an intervention when the power of the urge to binge overcomes them. They can allow themselves to experience their feelings so they can express them rather than feed them more food.

Sooner or later food loses its ability to dull the pain of unexpressed feelings. Turning to it or any other substance for solace is seeking your identity from the outside, where it can never be found. The form your addiction takes really doesn't matter. It's the content, namely your emptiness, that matters, that void you feel you have to fill up with someone or something outside of yourself to feel complete.

Hitting Bottom

Hitting bottom is that moment when food no longer alters your state of mind and you really feel the depths of your anguish. Reality glares like a spotlight on the truth of your situation, illuminating what you've been trying so hard to deny—that your life is unmanageable, that you're both helpless and hopeless and can find no way out of your pain short of dying.

No one else can measure that pain. It can't be calibrated by whether you have two hundred pounds to lose or twenty. If those extra pounds are making you miserable, damaging your self-esteem and your ability to cope with life, or if you're keeping your normal weight by secret vomiting, or if you're so thin people are alarmed while your mind is still telling you you're fat, the pain is all the same—unmeasurable. Only you know when you've taken all the pain you can stand.

Be glad you've hit bottom, because once you've arrived at that despairing place, you can change. Your chances for recovery are actually greater than those for people who don't feel desperate. There's a Zen saying,

"When the student is ready, the teacher appears." Once you've acknowledged you don't have the answer, you open yourself up to the possibility of seeking an answer elsewhere—one that *does* work. Hitting bottom isn't the end of the world. It's the anteroom to a new one. It's not a tragedy. It's an epiphany.

Getting Help

It may be no accident this book appeared in your life at this particular time. If you're ready to get help, you can determine what kind you need at the end of this chapter, where there is a quiz you can take. It will help you determine whether you're addicted to food. Going into treatment is the ultimate preparation for recovery, but that may not be possible for you in your present circumstances. I have written this book to serve as an alternative to treatment. If you commit yourself to following the steps laid out before you here, it will be the next best thing to experiencing a treatment center.

Merely reading this book, however, will not get you on the road to recovery. **"You can't think yourself into good acting, but can act yourself into good thinking."** My program requires you to take action, even before you believe it will work for you. In fact, the addict in you will really rebel at first, and do everything to convince you that your new attempt is just another failure on your part. But if you ignore the voice of that powerful disease within you that is causing you so much pain, and take the simple actions required by this program, I'm telling you now you *will* succeed. I did, and you can, too.

Fifteen years ago I weighed 340 pounds and was a full-blown alcoholic. I was a single parent with a high school diploma, three kids, and no future I could see for myself. At that crucial point in my life I had the great fortune to meet people who believed in me when I couldn't. Would you permit me to return the favor and believe in you?

Today, fifteen years in recovery, I am a psychologist with a Ph.D. I'm a pioneer in the field of eating disorders, I'm in seven Who's Who publications, a columnist for two counseling magazines, a director on the International Association for Eating Disorder Professionals, and am just opening up the fourth Janet Greeson's "A Place For Us", a center for the treatment of eating disorders. But most important, I am happy. My life is rich and full. I have many deep and meaningful relationships. I no longer live in that despairing state of isolation I knew when I was active in my disease. I'm a success story, and you can be one, too.

There's a psychotherapeutic principle I believe in, that you can't take a patient where you haven't been yourself. Because I am an alcoholic as well as a food addict, I know the needs of both and how they differ, I know the addiction from the inside out, and I attribute the high rate of success in our treatment centers to my once having been in the same situation my patients are in. Cross-addiction is more common than most people realize. Because so many alcoholics develop an addiction to food, especially sugar, while in recovery, it is beneficial to treat both addictions at once. **"Substituting one addiction for another is like changing chairs on the *Titanic*."** It's important addicts learn that early. Without the knowledge that they may substitute one addiction for another. Addiction is addiction. There is not any one that is not life threatening.

Treatment at Janet Greeson's "A Place For Us" consists of a 28-day program of three nutritionally balanced low-fat meals a day, abstinence from sugar, caffeine, white flour, and other mood-altering substances, exercise of up to an hour each day, cognitive groups, intensive, action-oriented group therapy, learning and enactment of social skills, and nightly attendance at Overeaters Anonymous, and other 12-Step programs. Much of the program at Janet Greeson's "A Place For Us" can be replicated by reading this book and participating wholeheartedly in its activities.

My treatment philosophy in this book reflects the particular needs of the food addict. Nearly all food addicts come into treatment voluntarily, desperate for help, whereas many people admitted into drug and alcohol treatment centers are required to do so by the courts, employers, or other authorities. Alcohol and drug addicts have often built up a false and very tough ego structure that must be broken down before they can get better. Food addicts have been so humiliated by their disease they don't need to undergo the breaking down of ego structures. More likely, they come in with low self-esteem, which they fill up with food. They see themselves in terms of externals—the roles they play in life of spouse, parent, son, daughter, employee—and when they enter treatment and can't play those roles or stuff their emptiness with food, they are terribly vulnerable. We treat them gently. We make them feel safe, warm, and loved. In that protective environment, with their regular lives in suspension, they are often able to make miraculous and permanent transformations.

My own attitudes toward healing have been greatly influenced by Gerald G. Jampolsky, MD, author of *Teach Only Love*. He writes, "Attitudinal healing recognizes a reality that is not connected to troubles, upsets, or even tragedies. That reality is love. Love is entered and assimilated only as our mind loses interest in either fighting against or succumbing to the miseries of life . . . The truth of love cannot be applied; it can only fill our hearts. Once this is done we will instinctively act in an appropriate way."

I have discovered this to be consistently true. It is the source of the miracles that happen at Janet Greeson's "A Place For Us" all the time. We focus on emotions, the internal emptiness, and the lack of boundaries, and all the rest follows. First the body responds, to the new way it's being fueled, and then the mind follows—not the judgmental, cynical, chaotic conscious mind, but the imprisoned spirit of the addict that yearns to be free. That responds to the new messages it is receiving and starts rattling its prison bars. By *doing*, not *thinking*, the body will set it free. Do you feel resistance in yourself to reading these words? That's your disease stirring. Take it along with you into these pages. It will never leave you, but after you've released your spirit, you can arrest the disease and put *it* behind bars, one day at a time.

In order to give up something you have needed as

desperately as your addiction, you must replace it with something else, for nature abhors a vacuum. If you don't want to be reading this with a Devil Dog in each hand by the second chapter, you must do more than think. Thinking has gotten you where you are now. Addicts of all kinds go in for magical thinking. They like to go to doctors who give them pills and tell them they're going to be okay. They can go into individual therapy and get stuck in the talking mode forever. But there is no magic to getting better. You have to *do* something. You have to change. How many people do you know who have been going to therapists twice a week for five, ten, fifteen, and even twenty years and are still miserable? I know the one-on-one process sometimes works. I also know it's not always the solution. You might gain some new awareness in years of therapy, but I don't know if insight is enough. Knowledge makes you smart but it doesn't necessarily give you recovery.

My philosophy of treatment is radically different from what most centers offer. We're about change more than just dealing with awareness and pain. Because food addicts are isolates, we stress the development of intimacy skills. Other treatment centers focus on past issues, but I believe people are going to deal with their pain anyway, and if our therapists focus on it alone, the patients still leave with the problem of feeling isolated, incapable of intimacy, and not knowing how to really live. We teach and get them to practice the basic social skills they may have forgotten, or if they grew up in a dysfunctional family, they may never have learned, so they can achieve the intimacy they desire.

The only time we deal with the past is when patients have important unfinished business, hurts that are blocking them and need to be expressed, particularly anything that has been kept a secret such as sexual or other forms of child abuse. **"You're only as sick as your secrets,"** and they are always an impediment to recovery. In order to build a new foundation for life, they have to be revealed, forgiven, and disposed of. I have found the incidence of childhood sexual abuse among food addicts far greater than in the average population. In fact, the figure is so high it makes me wonder whether there's a "funny uncle" in nearly every food addict's family closet. I have come to the conclusion that many food addictions develop because food is the only mood-altering substance readily available to children, and when they use it to help them over a trauma, it becomes a lifelong coping mechanism. The use of food as a reducer of childhood stress is nearly universal. When babies cry, what happens? They get a bottle.

When a patient has unfinished business, we deal with it in psychodrama and group therapy. In psychodrama the incidences of physical and emotional abuse, loss, and guilt over a past event are redramatized so the feelings of anger and pain surrounding them can be identified and expressed. A lot of people have never experienced that pain because they were afraid nobody was going to be there for them. Sometimes the experience is overwhelming, and they're afraid they're going to lose control, but the pain of those traumatic events must be reexperienced before healing can take place. You can't go around it, deny it, or back away from it. The only way out is through, with a therapist, a group, a buddy, or all three.

Patients go through the pain in a safe environment with people they trust, people they can count on to give them the support they need. People share secrets about their lives that no one else in the world knows. In the process their shared vulnerabilities bond them for life. Even if they don't carry on a relationship with each other physically, they remain bonded spiritually because they have assisted each other in a powerful healing process, a kind of emotional chemotherapy, exorcising destructive feelings they have been holding on to that have been making them ill all their lives.

Once they've identified their feelings, they need to learn to experience and express them to keep from exploding them in a binge or a purge. Addicts haven't learned how to trust their feelings or listen to their emotions. They haven't learned to take actions on their thoughts, not their feelings. A lot of addicted people don't even realize that feelings pass, that they don't have to own them forever.

Other than clearing up major issues of unfinished business, our psychotherapeutic approach is not to go back to day one to find out the root causes of behavior. There's not time for that in twenty-eight days. We focus on the feelings of here and now. Instead of concentrating on the behavior that the disease has caused, we work on creating new behavior, new identities, and new attitudes.

Too often people in therapy keep waiting for something to happen. I say you have to make it happen and get in touch with the energy that taking action releases. Then you can take that energy and go outside of yourself and feel a part of the universe, combining energies with others to create a sense of belonging. Knowing you're a part of something good and useful and making a contribution to it is what leads to recovery.

There's more resistance in the mind to getting well than there is in the body. Addicts have worked too hard for too many years reprogramming their minds to give it all up without a struggle, but if they don't think too much about what they need to do, they'll get there. The sickness that rages in food addicts' bodies is the direct result of what's going on in their heads, which are full of negative thoughts about themselves and others. Those thoughts are the bars that make up your prison. They need to be replaced with positive thoughts and action so the real you can be freed to have a life. Fortunately, the laws of physics are on our side: Everything in nature moves from a negative to a positive, but never the other way around. How many negative people attract you? Or do you gravitate toward those who feel good about themselves and others?

Changing negative thoughts to positive ones is called cognitive restructuring. For the mind to register a negative thought, it has to think it in a positive first. When it hears "Don't eat," the mind registers two sentences: first, "Eat," and then, "Don't eat." I believe it's better to say "Stay sober and go to meetings" than the traditional "Don't drink and go to meetings," because the mind registers "Drink" before "Don't drink." Most people don't even realize they have a choice about how they think and that knowledge is tremendously liberating. You can choose your thoughts but not your feelings. Feelings are reactions to thoughts.

There are only two things in life you can ever control: your thoughts and your behavior. You can't change your feelings; feelings just are. But you can change your response to them and then, like a miracle, the feelings will change without your doing anything about them. At the center we teach a "do-feel-believe" pattern of behavior change. Change the behavior whether you think it's going to work or not. **"Bring the body and the mind will follow." "Fake it till you make it."**—these slogans (they will appear frequently in this book) are the distilled word-of-mouth wisdom repeated over and over by millions of people in 12-step programs who for many years have been successfully helping each other change their destructive behavior patterns. Nobody knows who said them first, but they're repeated like a litany because they work.

As you participate in the treatment section of this book, you will also be engaged in cognitive restructuring. Even while you sleep your mind will be processing the change in thought processes, and your dreams will be like road maps on the journey to recovery. Detours don't get you there. Belief systems simply cannot be penetrated in a weekend or even a week-long seminar, no matter how inspiring the lecturer or how confrontational the technique. In fact, highly confrontational seminars can do great damage, especially to food addicts, who tend to have a fragile ego structure. On the other hand, many of the more loving and supportive encounter groups that were popular in the sixties and seventies were on the right track, but they didn't give people the tools to change. They failed because they didn't go far enough.

How to Make the Most of This Book

At this point you are probably thinking, this is all very fine for people who can afford to go into treatment, but what about me? You can apply much of what is done in treatment at home. Here's how:

Section Two of this book is divided into twenty-eight days. If you are an overeater, there is a weight-loss food plan designed to reorient your body to healthy eating, not take off a lot of pounds all at once, although you will definitely lose weight if you follow it. If you are bulimic or anorexic, there is a weight-maintenance and weight-gain food plan designed to reassure your body that you are now acting responsibly toward it.

Each day includes a classroom lecture in which new concepts will be explained, followed by workbook assignments for you to complete. There will also be positive affirmations and meditations for you to practice. Sample journal entries appear at the end of each day of treatment, describing what is seen, heard, felt and learned so you can identify with what might pertain to you. You will also be keeping your own journal to mark your progress through treatment. The twenty-eight days it takes to complete the program will be busy ones, and it will be necessary for you to find time to devote to it, for it will take your full involvement to leave the state of disease and enter the state of recovery.

You must read this book slowly—one day at a time for twenty-eight days—and participate 100 percent. If you read this book in two days, you cannot expect any results.

You Can't Do This Alone!

If you have unfinished business of your own, particularly issues of childhood abuse, it will block your recovery and I strongly urge you to seek therapy. Some mental health associations have a sliding-scale fee schedule, and you pay according to your income. On "Day Eleven" in the treatment section, I discuss "Choosing a Therapist." I suggest you read that section before you begin your search.

If you are fortunate not to have a lot of unfinished business in the way of your recovery, you still can't get there alone. Remember, food addiction is a disease of isolation. I highly recommend you follow the course of treatment with a buddy, someone you know who shares your problem, someone you feel close to and trust. Some of the workbook assignments require a partner, and it is also important to have someone to reach out to when the urge to act compulsively overwhelms you.

In addition, you will need to find 12-step meetings. Even if you and a buddy follow the workbook exercises to the letter, you still need the power of a group. In the years I have been in recovery I have known hundreds of food addicts, many of whom had struggled unsuccessfully with their addiction all their lives, who worked the steps of the program and were released of their insane craving for food. Why it happens is a question I can't answer. How it works is one I can, for it is a well-defined process that involves only one thing: changing your behavior in a way that will make you happy, joyous, and free. The process is simple but not easy. The simple part is the lifting of the craving for food, which is unquestionably a blessing, but it is not easy to restore a life that has been damaged by addiction. The progress there is slow, hard work, but the saying **"There are no failures in OA, only slow recovery"** is one I have found to be true.

You may balk at the idea of needing to belong to a group, but there's nothing to join. Twelve-step meetings require no membership, dues, or fees. They pass a basket at meetings to help meet the rent, but a voluntary contribution is the extent of the commitment anyone has to make.

Overeaters Anonymous groups are listed in most telephone directories, or you can call or write the national headquarters. Many lunch-hour meetings take place in business districts; other meetings are held in the evenings in churches or schools. You may be surprised to find out you've been passing a meeting place regularly and didn't even know it was there.

When people first start going to meetings, I tell them to shop around. They are run by addicts like yourselves, so you are bound to meet some people who are too much to bear! Some meetings are more loving than others, and a few are too rigid or judgmental for comfort. **"Take what you like and leave the rest."** If the first group you find doesn't give you what you need, keep looking until you find one that does. Some meetings tend to focus on the addiction and others tend to focus on recovery. I prefer the latter. I know more than enough about my addiction but never enough about recovery. Once you find a group that makes you feel at home, keep going back. When patients ask me, "How long do I have to go to meetings?" I tell them, "Until you want to go." When you start out, it's good to know the feeling of "have to go" will leave and you will want to go to the fellowship. We were not meant to live alone. Only the addict in you believes that, so it can continue to wield its power over you.

People who are born with endorphin deficiencies can become addicted to meetings, because being around loving, caring people raises their endorphin level. Their life is terrible, they feel awful, everything's going wrong, and someone suggests they go to a meeting. There they get an endorphin rush and feel immediately better, although they can't tell you exactly what was said or what happened to improve their mood. I wouldn't worry about becoming addicted to meetings, particularly if you're one of those born with an endorphin deficiency. To me, the benefits of the fellowship far outweigh any concern about whether people will become addicted to meetings because in themselves they fulfill a basic human need to be sociable.

You will probably find that after a few weeks of meetings, you will begin to crave them. Some people object to these 12-step programs as "just another addiction." My guess is that statement is either being made by a nonaddictive person or an addict in denial. Creating another craving to fill the void in the absense of food is essential until that void begins to be filled with the "real you."

You may also be one who objects to all the "God stuff," particularly if you were a victim of religious abuse in your childhood. The spirituality of a 12-step program has nothing to do with religion. If you are ready to accept the idea that your own power is not enough to cope with your addiction to food, you will soon discover that the power of the group is greater than your own. That can become the higher power you seek, and you need to go no further to find it. Once you identify with it, your own power is released. The experience is not mystical in any way. It's tangible. That is, it can be felt and needs no explanation or interpretation. After feeling bad for so long, even a few moments of this new joyfulness will keep you going until it grows. Just remember you're not responsible for the results. When you can let go of the outcome, I guarantee you it will turn out exactly as it's supposed to.

To me, spirituality is the positive energy you possess that has been blocked by your addiction. It is your own higher self. Instead of looking for some deity in the sky, I want you to go inside of yourself and get in touch with the good that lies within you. Did you ever see a baby you instantly liked? There are some babies I just don't take to, but then there are others whom I respond to with a smile because they are so completely in touch with the good within them. I like the baby even though it doesn't tell me I'm good-looking or nice or that it loves me. It's the baby's energy I'm experiencing, this joyous feeling of "there's absolutely nothing wrong with me." Babies can't tell you about it. You just sense it. It's as if they're saying, "Aren't I wonderful?" and of course they are, and you can feel the tremendous amount of energy behind that idea.

Or sometimes that energy is present in an adult who has died but you feel they are still with you in some way—their spirit stays with you and continues to nurture you as the years go by because they have had such a positive impact on your life. That's the kind of spirit I mean: not an invisible authority figure but the positive and constructive force that lies in all of us like buried treasure beneath a slag heap of negative and destructive thoughts. As my good friend Father Leo Booth puts it, "You can take the alcohol out of the alcoholic, but you're still left with the 'ick.'" Transcending the "ick" is what spirituality is all about.

Recovery is about healthy rituals that bind us to others. It's being connected to the world in a meaningful way. It's also being connected to the Real You within, who has been imprisoned by addiction. The revelation of who that really is does not come about by learning something new but by the uncovering of who you are by nature. The bright colors of autumn are present in the leaves all along, but they can't be seen until the chlorophyll departs through their veins and returns to the tree. Your natural brilliance is like that. It's in you already, concealed by whatever defenses you have used all these years to protect your vulnerability. The unveiling of that hidden beauty is painful, like all change, but that pain is quickly forgotten when you see the spectacular results.

I am often amazed to discover how many food addicts don't see their own beauty. Debbie, an anorexic you'll read about in this book, was a particularly attractive patient who came into my office one day to talk about an episode of the television show *Beauty and the Beast*. As I listened to her, it became obvious to me that she identified more with the character of the Beast than the Beauty! The lovely, warm, ebullient woman who stood before me saw herself as ugly and an outcast. It became obvious to me that Debbie's obsession to transform what she saw as a completely unacceptable body image had led to her eating disorder.

I then recalled how struck I had been by a television interview with Ron Perlman, who plays the beast in *Beauty and the Beast*. He talked quite emotionally about how he related to his character because he was obese as a child. When asked what it was like to be in love, he responded, "The end of loneliness." Here was someone who had gone from being unacceptable to incredibly acceptable, still relating to other people with the pain of the outcast. When I saw *Phantom of the Opera*, I was struck by the way the main character was transformed from a grotesque figure into someone who moved me to tears by the end of the play. I have come to believe these and other dramatizations, such as *Mask* and *The Elephant Man*, all about people who have been ostracized because they do not meet the prescribed standard of physical beauty, strike a deep chord in us. Everyone can identify with their pain because none of us feels acceptable, even the beauties.

It's helpful to remember that even the fortunate ones, whose good looks we may envy, are rarely happy about their bodies. How tragic it is that we all seem to buy into the media myth that how we look is who we are! In the end, what does our outward appearance really mean? A package can be wrapped very attractively and expensively, but how long can anyone remain interested in an unopened gift? After that overrated first impression has been made, what people really relate to is your energy, and if there is nothing radiating from within that attracts others, you can be gift-wrapped by Tiffany and it won't matter.

Getting real is what matters, the great relief of giving up all the false roles you thought you had to play to survive, to discover the joy of just being yourself and knowing it's all you need to be. Once you're real, you can be intimate with others. You can bond with them, and food will no longer be the focus of your life. Years ago if you had asked me who I was, I would have told you I was a housewife, a mother, a Brooklynite—I would have told you all different kinds of things about me or what I did, but all of them image. Today I would tell you I'm Janet, the caring person. The real me is loving and spontaneous and creative and attractive and sensual. I hope this book will help you reach beyond your image to find out who you really are. Most likely you don't even know who that is yet, but I can promise you, the person you've always wanted to be awaits you in recovery.

Not everyone has the courage to do what you're about to do, and I commend you for it. Be grateful for your pain, for it has gotten you this far. You're lucky. You're one of the chosen.

Workbook

ARE YOU A FOOD ADDICT?

You have an important choice to make. More important than what is happening around you is what is happening inside you. Answer the following questions honestly with a "yes" or a "no."

1. Have you had a weight problem for longer than five years? _____
2. Is there a history of obesity in your family? _____
3. Is there a history of depression or anxiety in your family? _____

4. Is there a history of alcoholism in your family? _____
5. Is there a history of drug abuse in your family? _____
6. Is food associated with good feelings in your family? _____
7. Does food make you feel good? _____
8. Do you ever get depressed about your weight? _____
9. Do you eat when you're not hungry? _____
10. Do you go on eating binges for no apparent reason? _____
11. Do you have difficulty concentrating or making decisions? _____
12. Do you plan secret binges? _____
13. Do you often feel sad, blue, irritable, or worried? _____
14. Do you ever have feelings of worthlessness? _____
15. Do you lack confidence in yourself? _____
16. Have you ever tried to lose weight by severely restricting your food intake? _____
17. Do you ever self-induce vomiting? _____
18. Do you often feel nervous and high-strung? _____
19. Have you ever lost interest or pleasure in usual activities, or have you had a decrease in your sex drive because of your weight? _____
20. Do you feel more tired than usual? _____
21. Have you wished yourself dead, attempted suicide, or feared dying? _____
22. Have you ever felt as if you didn't care anymore? _____
23. Do you feel depressed, guilty, or remorseful after overeating? _____
24. Do you become suddenly scared for no apparent reason? _____
25. Do you avoid or withdraw from others due to your weight or food intake? _____
26. Do you ever have spells of the blues, down in the dumps? _____
27. Are you experiencing sadness that doesn't seem to want to go away? _____

28. Do you see yourself a loser at times? _____
29. Do you have difficulty asking for help? _____
30. Do you ever feel like nothing you do matters? _____
31. Have you ever lied about your weight? _____
32. Do little annoyances get on your nerves and irritate you? _____
33. Do you feel as if you won't be able to stop eating certain foods once you start? _____
34. Do you have an intense fear of getting fat? _____
35. Have you missed days of work because of overeating, weight, or related illness? _____
36. Do you take things very personally? _____
37. Do you overcommit yourself? _____
38. Do you feel responsible and think you are responsible for other people, or another person's feelings, thoughts, actions, choices, wants, needs, well-being, lack of well-being? _____

If you answered "yes" to ten or more of the questions, you have an important choice to make. You can choose a new life for yourself, free of food addiction and depression. You can stop living to eat and start eating to live.

2

The First Step

Elaine

Only one light was on in the Peterson house. Everyone was asleep except Elaine, whose presence at the refrigerator around twelve-thirty was becoming a nightly occurrence. Over the weeks since she began making her nocturnal visits to the kitchen after the Johnny Carson show, the form that stood in the light of the open refrigerator door cast a shadow on the kitchen floor that grew and grew.

As soon as Johnny's smile began to fade from Elaine's television screen, it seemed her mind could no longer control her body. Cursing at herself under her breath, her feet carried her to the kitchen, her heart beat fast as if on the way to a clandestine love affair, and her whole being lusted for the contents of the refrigerator, every little tidbit she had been virtuously resisting all day and most of the night. For hours the container of rice pudding had been calling to her, joined by the three short ribs left over from dinner, swimming in her special barbecue sauce, and in the back of the bottom shelf where she had hidden it behind a loaf of bread, the last of the lemon meringue pie. It was only a sliver, but she had been obsessing on it all night.

In the early stages of Elaine's bingeing she had just eaten the contents of the leftover dishes. Then she began to cook extra so there would be more leftovers. Soon her little cache of late-night appetizers wasn't enough, and with a "What the hell, I've blown my diet now" attitude she made excuses to go to an all-night supermarket, ostensibly for cat food or scouring pads but really for popcorn, potato chips, packages of cookies and cakes, enough for a party.

Sometimes she managed to wait until she got home, and other times she started eating in the car. Afterward, she went to bed, leaden and appalled at what she was doing, filled with shame. But she couldn't stop.

One night, the car binge still didn't satisfy her and she went into the kitchen and cooked herself a grilled-cheese sandwich. Suddenly her husband was standing in the doorway.

"What's going on?" he demanded.

"Just getting a head start on tomorrow's cooking," she lied. He didn't challenge that, but there was a disdainful look on his face.

Her extra weight obviously turned him off sexually, for he kept his distance from her in and out of bed. That was the deepest hurt of all, and yet she was fully conscious of everything she was doing. Cliff was not a big man, and she knew her extra weight made him feel small, but still she couldn't help herself. One night, hoping the truth would act as a deterrent, she got the courage to step on the bathroom scale. She had gained thirty pounds in three months. It had taken her a year to lose them. She wept. Her solace was immediate: more food.

Elaine's late-night snacking had begun around the

time she was passed over for a promotion at work. She was assistant to the personnel director in a large insurance company and had worked hard for many years in her department, often taking on the responsibilities of others for which she rarely got credit. Still, she was sure her boss knew who did the bulk of the work in the office, and she was humiliated when a woman with half her experience and dedication had been promoted to the head of the department.

In the first few weeks of her nocturnal bingeing, no one even seemed to notice the fact that she was gaining weight, which she helped conceal by bringing out from the back of the closet some of the size-20 clothes she used to wear. The sight of them depressed her.

Elaine had been battling her weight since childhood. All the women in her family were overweight, as far back as her great-grandmother. When things had been going well in her life, she had won temporary battles with her weight. For a while in her twenties she had even been pencil slim. The size-12 clothes from those days also hung in the back of her closet, a reminder of what a year of constant sacrifice could do. But she had been happy then, close to her husband, and a mother of children who had not yet become problems. Now she couldn't get close to her husband, literally. Her stomach was in the way, and she seriously doubted whether she could ever put herself through the deprivation of a crash diet again.

Three months after Elaine's failure to be promoted, her twenty-five-year-old daughter Kathleen's marriage ended and she returned home. Elaine took her son-in-law's desertion personally, as if she had been rejected herself. In her depression, she started making stops at a 7-Eleven store on the way home from work, eating entire packages of cookies and throwing away the evidence before pulling into her driveway.

The next time she stepped on a scale, she weighed 190 pounds, more than she had ever weighed in her life. That frightened her. For a week she managed to control her bingeing and was just starting to feel good about herself when, gathering together clothing to take to the dry cleaners, she found something in her husband's jacket pocket that plunged her back into her despair. It was a note that began "Darling" and ended "All my love, Suzanne," and in between was a plea that their affair had to end. When Elaine handed her husband the note, he was full of remorse and begged her forgiveness, insisting the affair had already ended. She didn't speak to him for days. One night he tried to make love to her and she shoved him away. How could he even try to touch her after cheating on her with another woman?

Now she had a good excuse to eat, she told herself, and she did so with a vengeance. When her weight went over 200 pounds, she told herself it didn't matter. Nothing mattered. As the weeks went by, her husband worked late almost every night at the office, and she told herself she didn't care whether he was really working or continuing his affair. When he crawled into bed at night, she always pretended to be asleep. Then she would lie awake wondering whether the fragrance she smelled on him was after-shave or a woman's cologne.

Before her life started unraveling, Elaine had a lot of acquaintances, although not many close friends. She was active in her church and her block association, and she thought of herself as being well liked by a lot of people, but when in her depression she began to withdraw from the world, her telephone stopped ringing. None of her so-called friends even bothered to find out if she was all right, and that filled her with despair, thinking back on all the phone calls she had made to people in her community just to check up on them and say hello. Several years before, the family had actually gone to the expense of putting in another line because she was on the telephone so much. Now when she returned home after being away for several hours and the digit on her answering machine still registered zero, she would sit by the telephone and weep.

The only person who kept calling was Margaret, a woman she had met in Weight Watchers. One day Margaret called her and offered to drive her to a meeting that night. Elaine said sweetly, "I tried Weight Watchers with you before, remember? It just didn't work for me."

"I don't go there anymore," said Margaret. "I go to a

new meeting, at the Civic Center, and it has really been working for me. Please come just once and try it."

Elaine begged off. She was not in the mood to start a new diet.

Elaine started having difficulty getting up in the morning and was running out of excuses for being late at work. She used up her sick days and then her vacation days. Finally, her department head called her in and said in a concerned voice, "Are you having difficulties at home?" Elaine burst into tears, hating herself for crying in front of this woman who had gotten the promotion that should have been hers.

The department head said she would be allowed to continue in her present position if she saw the staff psychologist. At first Elaine was furious that she had to confide in a total stranger in order to keep her job, but after a few weeks she found herself more and more willing to open up and talk about her problems. Nevertheless, the bingeing went on with a vengeance.

One afternoon, on the way home from her therapist, she stopped at a shopping mall to get her daughter a birthday present. Waiting in line at the cash register with a blouse she had picked out, she stared at the figure of a heavy woman who was wearing the same dress she was, and who looked very familiar. Then to her horror she realized she was staring at herself in a three-way mirror and quickly looked away. The sight of her bulging hips and the hugeness of her backside stayed in her memory for days, but it didn't keep her from bingeing. It seemed the bigger she was the more invisible she became.

Elaine ran into Margaret at the supermarket one day and she could tell her friend was shocked to see how much weight she had gained. Margaret grabbed her arm and said, "I heard about this place in Daytona Beach, Florida. Someone I know from my meeting just came back from there and has wonderful things to say about it. It's a treatment center for eating disorders."

Elaine laughed gaily. "Thanks for your concern, but you just don't understand. If I was away from my job for a few weeks I wouldn't have a job to come back to!"

Then one night, standing once again in the mesmerizing light of the open refrigerator door and eating from a bottle of olives, she blanked out as olive by olive the contents of the jar disappeared down her throat. The next thing Elaine knew, she was running to the downstairs bathroom where she threw up everything in her stomach.

Lying in bed that night, careful not to touch her husband, she realized to her horror that throwing up was the only way out and that she was going to take it, in spite of her hatred of the act. A bottle of olives apparently did the trick. She discovered other foods and avoided the ones that were hard to bring up. Popcorn was a nightmare, but ice cream was a good foundation. Other nights when the food wouldn't come up by itself, she used a drinking straw. Each time she went to the cupboard to get the box of straws, she told herself her shameful secret couldn't go on.

One night, listening to hear whether she had awakened anyone upstairs (it was hard to throw up quietly), she experienced a revelation that sent a shudder through her entire body. As if looking down from above, she saw herself kneeling before the toilet bowl in the dead of night, knees clutching the morgue-cold porcelain, keeping her hair out of the water in the bowl with both hands, and said out loud, "You've got to get help."

Tears flowed at the sound of her words. Still caught in the power of that moment of truth, she went straight to the telephone and called Margaret.

"Sorry to call so late," Elaine said, for a change not even pretending to be cheerful. "What's the name of that treatment center?"

Tony

Tony was thirty-five and the president and chief executive officer of his family-owned tool-and-die business. He had won that position in a battle with his older brother and a cousin, outwitting them by gaining the support of his father, who wanted to retire, and the outside shareholders. In the process, the entire family had taken sides, relationships were sundered, and some swore they would never speak to him again because of all the enmity he had caused. But Tony knew he had done the right thing. Had the other side won, the family business would have been sold against his father's wishes to the highest bidder. Tony vowed that would happen only over his dead body.

By the time the dust had settled, Tony had gained twenty pounds. It was a mystery to him how he had gained the weight. It had come over him like a sneak attack.

Right after he had been installed as CEO, another crisis hit. His competitors in the tool-and-die business attempted a hostile takeover of the firm. After eight months in a state of siege, Tony once again managed to keep the business in the family, but it owed over $250,000 in lawyers' fees and had spent millions refinancing. Tony had to let some employees go and do some major bottom-line readjustments, but in the end, the business was more fit than ever. He had gotten rid of some dead weight and some real troublemakers in the process.

Whan that crisis was resolved, Tony stepped on the scale one morning and found out he had put on another twenty pounds. He now weighed 240, more than he had ever weighed even in his football-playing years in college when he could eat all he wanted. Tony had never been slim, but no one had ever called him fat. "Beefy" was the word people used to describe him. Now when he looked in the mirror, he had to conclude that "fat" was the only word that fit. His clothes certainly didn't. In fact, he had to go out and spend a lot of money on a new wardrobe.

Tony had a secretary, Estelle, who had been with him for ten years. Her loyalty was such that he tolerated listening to her advice, which became more frequent concerning his weight gain. He gave up lunches for a week and lost a few pounds, which kept her off his case for a while. Tony didn't think his current problem with food was anything he couldn't handle. With the year he'd just been through, he figured it was a wonder he hadn't turned to more than just food. He knew men who popped pills, snorted cocaine, and drank three-martini lunches to handle the kind of pressure he'd been under.

Then, just when things were settling down and he was thinking about taking a vacation, his wife was diagnosed as having cancer. She had a mastectomy just before Thanksgiving. By New Year's, Tony weighed 280.

And still he kept gaining. He began wondering whether there was something wrong with his metabolism. His wife started buying his clothes in shops with names like Majestic Male, where shirts started at $50. His secretary continually criticized his eating habits. Finally he stopped giving her his lunch orders and called the restaurants himself, directing the delivery boy to bring his meals straight into his office. But one day his secretary waylaid two shopping bags of Chinese food and brought them into him herself.

"Is all this for you?" she said with a shocked look on her face.

"I didn't have time for breakfast," he said angrily. "Set up a conference call for me, will you?"

After the conference call was over, he looked down at the empty cartons of Chinese food on his desk and had no idea what had been in any of them. He had apparently inhaled the food without tasting it and had no recollection whatsoever of the act. That scared him, and annoyed him, too. Here he was, putting on all this weight and not even enjoying his food.

Tony had always liked to eat, and food was an important part of any family gathering. Both his parents had to watch their weight, and Tony had been on diets intermittently most of his adult life, managing to keep his eating under control enough to look decent in a business suit. An overweight CEO was asking for trouble. People would wonder whether his business was out of control, too. But not even the threat of losing his shaky hold over the business could keep him from eating too much.

The family squabble intensified when his brother-in-law did a shocking thing. He left Tony's sister and moved in with a woman half his age. Tony was very close to his sister, but he had never cared much for his brother-in-law, particularly after he came into an inheritance, invested heavily in the company, and was now a major stockholder. To make matters worse, Tony's sneaky older brother was taking advantage of the enmity between them and cozying up to Tony's brother-in-law, which made Tony very nervous. When he heard from his secretary that they and another rival had taken some of the important outside stockholders to a three-hour lunch at a very fancy restaurant, he stuffed down his worry with an entire pizza.

Usually Tony did his heavy eating during the day, but as he gained weight, it became difficult for him to get to sleep, and insomnia drove him to eating at night, too. It frightened him to be so out of control with his food. He had to be in control of things. Nothing in his life seemed to be on solid ground anymore. Everything was shifting.

He started sleeping in his recliner in the living room. The extra weight put pressure on his lungs and made it difficult for him to breathe lying flat in bed. He would settle in front of the TV with his treats all around him and fall asleep with the television on for a night-light, waking up near dawn to the empty chatter of a 1930s movie. Then he'd turn off the TV and drift back to sleep until his wife called him in the morning.

She was unhappy that he didn't come to bed at night.

"I just can't fall asleep in a bed," he said. For no reason she burst into tears.

Then she complained he didn't spend enough time with his kids. His son was doing poorly in school. Tony yelled at her, then apologized.

It was all getting to be too much for him to handle—the pressures of his business, worrying about his wife, feeling guilty about neglecting his kids, feeling sorry for his sister and angry at his brother. When he had to go to California for a business trip, he was glad to get away and stayed an extra week, thinking of it as a vacation. But he spent most of the time on the telephone, putting out fires back home. He returned more exhausted than when he had left and carrying another ten pounds of fat. It seemed to be literally leaping onto him these days. He swore he could pass through a dining room and gain weight by merely smelling the food.

One night late in January he woke up with severe palpitations in his chest. He was sure it was a heart attack. His wife heard him crying out and called an ambulance. As he lay strapped to a cot in the ambulance while it careened through the streets, siren screaming, a voice inside him said quietly, "You're going to die if you keep this up."

His wife held his hand all the way to the hospital, smiling and stroking his face with one hand and wiping the tears with the other.

"You'll be fine," she kept saying.

He was diagnosed in the emergency room as being morbidly obese. That word "morbidly" chilled him. He had not experienced a heart attack, but that could easily happen, the cardiologist warned him. His cholesterol was dangerously high. A low-fat, no-salt diet was mandatory.

After a few days' bed rest Tony returned to work, vowing to cut out all lunches. His secretary asked to see him before he bit into his first Danish. She handed him a pamphlet.

"What's this?" he said.

"I want you to read about where you're going," she said firmly. "I've cleared your calendar. Your insurance covers the full twenty-eight days."

"You're fired," he said.

"Fire me when you get back," his secretary replied, and then Tony remembered the way the siren had sounded from within the ambulance.

"All right," he sighed, "I'll fire you when I get back."

Jean

Jean had not always had her gorgeous figure. She spent a painful adolescence in Chubby Department clothes before she started getting tall. By college she was slim, but constantly dieting, and long-limbed, a real Southern beauty queen. After winning a local beauty contest, she dropped out of college in her junior year to become a model, over her minister father's strong objections. At first she modeled in an Atlanta bridal salon. Then, after dropping twenty pounds, she broke into print work. Photographs of her appeared in ads in several bridal magazines.

Jean's career came to a halt at the age of twenty-two when she married a television producer ten years her senior. Now Jean wanted to stay home and be a model wife. Besides, she was sick of dieting to stay underweight for the cameras. She had been attracted to her husband because he was a bit on the wild side like herself. They moved to Los Angeles and had parties for weekends on end. He introduced her to cocaine, which she liked a lot better than alcohol because it didn't have any calories. Like everything in her life, she did it to excess. The marriage was tumultuous. The newlyweds even fought at parties. He cheated on her and she cheated on him in retaliation. After two years she had had enough and moved back to Atlanta. She used her alimony settlement to buy a condo in a luxury skyscraper, got a ten-to-six job as a photographer's assistant, and did some modeling on the side, although at twenty-four she was already over the hill in the fashion business.

Jean couldn't afford cocaine on her salary, but alcohol sufficed. She had an affair with her boss. He left his wife and moved in with her, and her Los Angeles–style party life resumed on a lesser scale. Gone were the punch bowls of giant shrimp and the freebasing, but Jean's new lover also believed that nothing was much fun if it wasn't done to excess.

Several months of vodka sours resulted in a weight gain of ten pounds, which thrust Jean into a panic state. She envisioned herself back in the Chubby Department. Sick of dieting, she found there was an easy way out. She just went into the bathroom, stuck three fingers down her throat, and threw up. She had had a college roommate who did it. She had also taken laxatives to keep down the absorption of calories, and Jean tried them, too, and she was surprised to find she could even get hooked on laxatives.

By her twenty-fifth birthday, Jean thought she had stabilized her life pretty well. She could binge and purge and drink and still stay slim, and nobody needed to know how she did it. She was madly in love with her live-in photographer and was pretty sure he was going to divorce his wife and marry her. Then she could quit her job and be a full-time wife again, this time for good.

Shortly after her twenty-fifth birthday, Jean got a frantic middle-of-the-night telephone call from her mother. Her father had suffered a massive heart attack and wasn't expected to live. Jean rushed to the airport in a driving rainstorm, praying to a deity she hadn't been on speaking terms with for many years that her father wouldn't die before she got to his bedside. Her failure to please him would then be complete. She would have disappointed him up to the last possible moment.

But her father didn't die. He rallied miraculously, and by the time Jean arrived at the hospital he was holding court in his hospital room with his wife, children, and grandchildren around his bed as if it were a throne.

Her father had been saved by his iron constitution. He was a powerful man in every way, the oldest son of a wealthy landowner, minister of the largest church in town, and influential in the lives of everyone in his family and many in his community. Handsome, charming, and tyrannical, he ruled by whim and was constantly cutting people out of his will or putting them back in. Jean and her sister secretly referred to him as Big Daddy.

Although Jean loved her father, she also hated him. He had a way of making her feel humiliated and was constantly comparing her to her sister, Janet, who was five years older and couldn't be more upstanding and responsible. Janet had two perfect little girls, ages eight and six. The only thing her sister had failed to do was stay married. Ralph, her third husband, had come with her on the emergency, and it was obvious they weren't getting along so well either.

Uncle Joe, her mother's favorite brother, gave Jean a ride home from the hospital. He was also staying at her parents' house. Although everyone else in the family thought Uncle Joe was lots of fun, Jean always felt awkward and uncomfortable in his presence, and she didn't like being alone in the car with him.

That night Jean went to bed in her childhood room. For hours she lay unable to get to sleep. Her father's close call had stirred up old fears of being lost or waking up alone in a strange place. When she finally drifted off to sleep, the fears invaded her dreams. The next thing Jean knew, she was sitting up in bed in a state of terror, her covers clutched to her chest, wondering what she had been dreaming that would make her shout out loud. Then she saw someone standing in the doorway.

"What's the matter, honey?" asked her Uncle Joe.

"Nothing, just a bad dream," said Jean. Her sister and husband were sleeping in the next room. That comforted her, but it took a long time before she got back to sleep. The next morning she was in a fog of depression that would not lift. A lot of parishioners came to the house, many of them bringing food. Jean ate four brownies and threw them up. While she was lying down, she heard her mother and sister in sotto voce conversation in the next room and caught the words "anorexic" and "vomiting again." There were no secrets in her father's house. Jean wondered how soon she could make plans to fly back to Atlanta.

Three days after her arrival, Jean had a fight with her mother over nothing at all. She told her sister her mother didn't like Jean's attitude or something. Then her sister got involved trying to patch things up. Jean decided she had to get out of her parents' house before she lost her mind. She stopped off at the hospital and saw her father, who was in great spirits, and then took a taxi to the airport without saying good-bye. She didn't care what they thought of her. They had one good daughter, she told herself. That was more than a lot of families had.

She couldn't wait to get back to the comfort of her own apartment and her boyfriend, who would console her and tell her she had done the right thing. She couldn't get the key to turn in the lock fast enough. The first thing she thought when she opened her front door was that they had been robbed. The VCR was gone, and the exercise bike. Then she found the note. Her lover had moved back in with his wife. She called all her friends and they came over to console her. Then she went on a three-day bender.

Jean now had serious money problems. Her photographer lover could hardly keep her on as his assistant now that he was back with his wife. She went to a new modeling agency and the booking agent was impressed by her portfolio, although he said she looked a lot older than her photographs. But her legs were still in good shape, and he said he would send her to a lingerie catalog house once she dropped ten pounds. Jean was euphoric, but the good news still wasn't money in the bank.

She hated the idea of taking in a roommate, and with great reluctance she called her father and asked for a loan. He laughed. "A loan? Since when have you ever paid me back? How much do you need this time?"

After that phone call she drank half a bottle of Johnnie Walker Red, straight shots.

Jean's usual dieting routine was to starve herself during the week and binge and purge on the weekends. After a few days, she discovered she no longer had the willpower to do that and was bingeing and purging every day. It was simple to do if she was drunk enough. The ten pounds came off without difficulty, and her agency started sending her out. Photographers liked her portfolio, but when they did test shots, they didn't call her back. Her lifestyle was beginning to show up in the photographs. She took off another five pounds, hoping that would make her more attractive, and tried to keep her bingeing under control, but as soon as Jean tried to keep anything under control, she lost what little she had.

After a month of making the rounds, she had not secured a single booking and her money was running out. Jean found a roommate, a quiet, kind social worker, and then sought out an employment agency. The first thing the interviewer asked her to do was take a typing test.

"I don't know how," said Jean.

"I can't send you out on a receptionist job without typing," she said. "Can you file?"

After three days of sticking little slips of paper in file drawers of a wall of floor-to-ceiling cabinets in a law firm, nearly fainting many times from bending down and straightening up, Jean decided it was time to die. She could no longer keep any food down and couldn't think of a single reason why she should remain alive. It was a Friday. Her roommate was gone for the weekend and wouldn't be back until late Sunday night. She returned home, closed the draperies, and lay down on her couch. She was so weak, giving up the ghost would be easy. All she had to do was lie there long enough. The phone kept ringing but she let her machine answer it, turning down the volume so she couldn't hear who was calling. She lay there all weekend, going in and out of consciousness. Once, dreaming of her boyfriend, she reached out to answer the phone, thinking it might be him. When she heard her roommate's voice, she started to cry.

"What's the matter?" her roommate said. "Are you sick? I'm coming home to help you."

Jean woke up to a room of buzzing voices, a friend packing her things, her roommate on the telephone making arrangements with a hospital.

Finally she hung up the phone and said, "Everything's been arranged. I'll drive you to the airport. Can you get these clothes on yourself or do you need help?"

"Where am I going?" she said.

"To Orlando."

Jean felt instantly better and managed to dress herself in a fog of dizziness and confusion. She was going to Florida. Disney World. That was nice. January in Florida.

Jean left for Janet Greeson's "A Place For Us" on a "snack" flight. Greedily she ate the two packs of peanuts the beverage-cart hostess handed her along with a Bloody Mary. When the snack trays came around, she didn't turn hers down, although she knew the food would be awful, and wolfed down the oversalted fake deli ham and cheese on rye, drank another Bloody Mary, ate the frosted cupcake, and then ran into the bathroom and threw up. One last binge, she figured. That made things nice and symmetrical. All she knew about rehab centers was they took away your drugs, cleaned you out, and sent you home. She could use that.

Wiping her face with a dampened paper towel, she peered at herself in the greenish light of the airplane bathroom, jerking and weaving with the sudden motions of the aircraft, and thought of how bizarre her life had become. The face that stared back at her was scarcely hers. Was this Jean the Prom Queen, Miss Runner-up, who was going to make it big in modeling and go on to the movies? She managed a cynical smile, thinking about her destination, and remembered what her mother had said about Uncle Joe the last time he went to dry out. He'd hit bottom, she'd said.

"You've hit bottom," she told the strange face in the mirror, watching her lips form stiffly around the words. "Nice going. You've hit bottom at forty thousand feet."

A driver in a white stretch limo picked her up at the airport. Jean smiled. Janet Greeson's "A Place For Us" did things in style. The limo driver chatted as she drove through the flatlands. Jean rolled down the window and breathed in the warm, moist air.

"My friend went through the program. It changed his life," the driver said. Jean smiled wanly. She didn't want to change her life. She just wanted to get well.

"No, really, dearie. It's true. I pick the patients up at the airport and I bring them back. I see what they're like before and after and I'm telling you, you won't believe the difference in yourself twenty-eight days from now."

The limo driver smiled at her, not a pasted-on smile but a genuine smile that went up into his eyes. For no reason at all Jean started to cry.

The Addictive Personality Profile

The following are characteristics of the addictive personality. Put a check by the ones with which you identify:

_____ Emotional extremes: You don't know anger, you know rage; you don't know fear, you know panic; you don't know pleasure, you know euphoria. With you it's all or nothing.

_____ Need for intensity: You relate to feelings, not facts, you crave excitement, you thrive on chaos.

_____ Need for immediate gratification: You want what you want when you want it and you want it now.

_____ Extreme thinking: You are either all wrong or you don't make mistakes. A situation is either black or white but never gray.

_____ Lack of identity: You need externals to

feel alive. You must always be doing something, and you overidentify with whatever it is.

_____ Lack of boundaries: You don't know where you end and someone else begins.

_____ Lack of moderation: Whatever you do, you overdo. If something works, taking more of it will work better. You have a pattern of playing at cards for hours, or at sports until you drop from exhaustion.

_____ Overreaction: You overreact to things outside of you and underreact to things inside of you.

_____ People pleasing: You are always looking for approval from others because you can't give it to yourself.

_____ Perfectionism: If you can't do it perfectly, you won't do it at all.

_____ Inability to express feelings: Most of the time you feel numb.

_____ Low self-esteem: You never feel you're good enough.

_____ Attraction to pain: You are compelled to seek out potentially harmful situations and company.

_____ Assumption: You make assumptions about what others feel rather than ask, then act as if that feeling is real.

_____ Projection: You fantasize about what will happen and are surprised when it doesn't turn out the way you imagined.

_____ Isolation: You feel as if you don't belong anywhere.

_____ Judgmental attitude: You are constantly judging and defending both yourself and others.

_____ Need for excitement: If you create enough chaos in your life, you don't have to look at what's really going on.

_____ Poor impulse control: Once you get an idea in your head, you can't rest until you act on it; once you start something, you can't stop until it's finished.

_____ Poverty mentality: You worry there won't be enough of what you crave.

_____ Supersensitivity: All your life people have told you that you are too sensitive, that you overreact to things.

3

Orientation to a New Life

If you follow the food plan, exercise between one-half to one hour each day, attend at least three meetings of Overeaters Anonymous a week, and make a full commitment to yourself in the workbook section to change your mental attitude and behavior patterns, you will be a different person by the time you finish reading this book. It will be a gift to yourself that will keep on giving, and the next best thing to a treatment program.

Menus: It Is What You're Eating

The food philosophy at Janet Greeson's "A Place For Us" is simple: three high-fiber, low-fat meals a day, including foods from the four basic groups: meat, milk, and dairy; fruit; vegetables; and grain. Each of these food groups is represented at each meal to keep craving at a low level. One of the comments we hear most frequently from our patients is that the meals are satisfying. Because protein from red meat sources is hard on the kidneys and high in fat, the emphasis is on chicken and fish. Much research has been done on the connection between addiction and nutrition, and we have found that a high-protein diet, use of nutritional supplements, especially amino acids, and the elimination of all mood-altering substances, particularly white sugar and white flour, works best to help eliminate cravings as well as get the addict's body back in tune. According to James Shanks, D.O., whose specialty is the field of addictionology, the body processes white flour molecularly, the same way as sugar.

Refined sugars and white flour are linked to depression and mood swings, triggering the compulsion to binge in the same way alcohol does in the alcoholic. Refined sugars include honey, corn syrup, dextrose, and fructose. One expert I know calls these forms "sugar in drag." They have already been predigested, that is, broken down from a multiple to a single sugar molecule that is similar to the alcohol molecule. Complex sugars are present in fruit, vegetables, legumes, nuts, seeds, and whole grains, which provide all the carbohydrates you really need. They break down slowly in the digestive process and do not give the "rush" that triggers craving.

Binge foods are generally high in carbohydrates. Habitual bingeing releases large amounts of insulin, which stimulates the appetite ever further, prolonging the binge, and promotes the storage of the additional calories as fat. If you are a sweet binger, you can now understand why you can't stop after one; your body is conditioned to respond with a rush of insulin, resulting in uncontrollable hunger. In order to get your body to believe in you again, we take you off this cunning and powerful substance that has been acting like a drug in your system. Treating certain foods as mind-altering substances is the first step in real recovery for a food addict.

I recommend caffeine be eliminated because it, too, is a drug that separates mind from body, causing you to be in an altered state. Because it dilates the small blood vessels, they will contract during caffeine withdrawal, resulting in the headaches that are common during the first week of treatment. They will pass after a few days, as will the craving for caffeine. Substitute decaf coffee for a psychological lift, but don't apply this rigidly. Remember, rigidity is part of the addiction.

Pretty soon your body will begin to regulate itself without the need for artificial jolts of energy provided by these powerful and insidious drugs, sugar and caffeine. You will be amazed to discover how much of your mood swings, depression, and anxiety has been caused by the habitual ingesting of these drugs.

Two food plans are presented in this program: one for people who want to lose weight, and the other for those who want to maintain or gain weight. The weight-loss food plan is higher in protein so you won't feel so hungry between meals, accompanied by a lot of high-fiber vegetables and two servings of fruit a day. You may also have three servings of low-fat milk a day if you wish. You will get grain three times a week as well as at breakfast in the form of a cereal. A lot of people binge on grains, so we minimize them at first to avoid setting up cravings that will trigger one. Once your weight starts coming off, you can incorporate more grain into your food plan.

The calorie consumption per day for the weight-loss menu is between 1,000 and 1,300 calories, depending on whether milk is being drunk. Weight-loss patients can also write in items such as baked fish, diet dressing, cottage cheese, and yogurt. I don't recommend a diet lower than a thousand calories a day because you're not likely to get the vitamins and minerals you need on less than that. Patients also take a multivitamin each morning.

The average weight loss the first week is six to fifteen pounds. Much of that is usually water. Weight loss in the following weeks will usually be less dramatic, but it will be stabilized and mostly fat. How much weight people lose during treatment is not stressed (patients are weighed once a week and I recommend you do the same), and the amount lost varies a great deal. I've seen people lose as much as thirty pounds and as little as four during the course of treatment. Remember that rapid weight loss may do wonders for your state of mind, but it's hardly ever permanent. We'd rather see you lose negative thoughts, pent-up anger, unexpressed grief, and harmful defense mechanisms during the twenty-eight days of treatment than a whole lot of weight. That will come off slowly and permanently in recovery.

Bulimics who don't need to lose weight and anorexics are put on a food plan of 1,800 or more calories a day to maintain or gain weight. It includes more grains, plus a list of cottage cheese, plain yogurt, green beans, chickpeas, baked fish, peanut butter, baked potato, brown rice, chunk tuna, and whole wheat bread. Anorexics also get high-protein snacks between meals of sandwiches, crackers and cheese, yogurt, and fruit. Contrary to the latest opinions by nutritional experts, our diabetic patients are refined-carbohydrate sensitive and seem to do better on Janet Greeson's "A Place For Us" food plan.

Weight gain for anorexics and bulimics is very small, if any. Their metabolism has been lowered because they've been surviving on so few calories. Their bodies have developed a famine mentality, take the additional calories, and turn them into fat to store for later use. It takes a while before structured exercise rebuilds their depleted muscle and organ tissue. People who resort to surgical intervention, such as having their stomachs tied or filled with a balloon, also undergo a change in basal metabolism. Lean body mass (muscle) is usually lost. Each time they lose fat, the body responds by holding on to the stores it has and cutting down on the amount of energy expended while increasing appetite. It's no wonder some anorexics complain of feeling fat—they do have a higher percentage of body fat.

Fasting causes a loss of protein in the form of lean body mass, and when anorexics and overeaters start to eat again after a fast, they fill up with fat, not protein and muscle. The only way to build up lean body mass after fasting is by exercise coupled with good nutrition. Some physicians treating anorexics refrain from letting them exercise, but they really need to be exercising in order to build up their lean body mass.

We used to give the old-fashioned basal metabolism

test using a face mask to determine how many calories a patient should be eating per day in order to lose or sustain weight, but this test is now done by a computer analysis called the Electroliprogram, and it is much more accurate than the old method. The test is remarkably simple. A device placed on the wrist for a mere fifteen seconds determines not only basal metabolism rate but also pounds and percentage of body fat, pounds and percentage of lean body mass, pounds and percentage of body water, and recommendations regarding loss of body fat.

And that's just the beginning! The computer then spews out a daily food plan with caloric recommendations based on the level and intensity of exercise the patient has selected. It breaks down each meal into kinds of proteins, carbohydrates, and fats that should be eaten and in what amount. It spells out fruits, vegetables, and grains that can be exchanged in making carbohydrate selections, and what kind of beverages may be used. It even gives an exercise prescription, complete with kind, duration, and calories burned for each day of the week.

These computer analyses are new, but because of their accuracy they are being adopted with great enthusiasm by many doctors, nutritionists, and treatment centers.

Twenty-eight days of regulated eating will result in a resumption of trust on the part of your body. It becomes convinced you're going to nourish it properly. Slow weight loss or gain, plus daily exercise, will actually raise your metabolism rate—as long as you don't skip meals. If you forsake breakfast and lunch, your body will once again stop trusting you and defend itself by craving food all night. Since your metabolism decreases about 10 percent when you sleep, it's the worst possible time to be consuming extra calories.

Remember, if your metabolism rate is low, don't lose heart! You can increase it by eating three meals a day, exercising regularly, and losing weight gradually.

You've Got to Move That Body

The exercise program at Janet Greeson's "A Place For Us" is geared to the physical condition of the patient. We recommend aerobic exercise—large muscle, continuous motion in the form of walking, jogging, or running. People who are twenty to thirty pounds overweight exercise up to an hour each day by walking. That builds up stamina without causing them injury, which a more stressful form of exercise could do.

If you are not exercising regularly now, I'd like to get you into the habit of walking every day. It's a form of exercise that can be done anywhere and can be incorporated easily into a daily schedule of activity. Your goal should be to walk a minimum of twenty miles by the end of the twenty-eight days. The speed at which the patients in treatment walk is monitored by a nurse, taking regular pulse rates and educating them as to what a safe target pulse rate is for their age and weight. You can learn to monitor your own.

Target heart rate is figured out by the following formula: 200 minus your age, multiplied by 60 percent, then divided by six. That's how many heartbeats you should strive for in a ten-second period. Later, when you are more fit, you can increase your heart rate by multiplying by 70–85 percent. Four or five beats over your target means you should slow down. If you don't have a pedometer, you can gauge your distance: A mile is covered in a fifteen-to-twenty-five-minute fast-paced walk. It takes six weeks before you will really start to feel the benefits of daily exercise. Your body will become more shapely, you will feel less stressed, and your stamina will increase.

People who are not severely overweight can elect to jog, run, or take aerobics for their exercise period. At the center we have added a new form of exercise, dance, which the patients love—jazz, ethnic, and social dancing, even dirty dancing. Many overweight people have yearned to learn these dances but have been too intimidated by their size to join a dance class. Other forms of exercise we recommend are swimming (it slows down the burning of fat but it does burn the calories), the minitrampoline, and rope skipping. Be sure you have good shoes if you choose the latter to protect your Achilles tendons. Frequency recommended is four to seven days a week, every day if sedentary, beginning with twenty to thirty minutes and progressing to an hour. Intensity is determined by monitoring the pulse for your target rate.

Treadmills have the highest percentage of success of any exercise machine, that is, people will stay with the treadmill longer than any other machine. I think it's because they can do other activities while using it, such as reading or watching television.

In treatment we keep the exercise time to an hour because anything longer than that makes people hungry. It will also work off emotions that should be taken to group.

Ground Rules for Change

BREAKING ISOLATION

People who seek help for an eating disorder are often in advanced stages of isolation. Their relationship with food seems to be their only rewarding experience. The loneliness that is felt is so profound nothing can fill it up but a substance to numb the emptiness, and food addicts do such a thorough job of withdrawing from family and friends, they are convinced it is they who have been shut out by others. Their expertise in guessing how others feel and think about them and their obsession about rejection only enhances their isolation, making it difficult for them to reach out and ask for help.

When they come into treatment, they have often lost the ability to take the first step in communicating with others. Most of their conversations are light. People-pleasers have highly developed social skills as far as talking to others and are externally oriented. Their conversations are more listening or about other people. They remain on the surface of their ability to express themselves because they don't have the intimacy skills of sharing who they really are, what they're about, and what their needs are.

Then there are the isolates. Lacking the social skills of the people-pleasers or just too afraid to take the risk of rejection, they remain in their rooms where they read, watch television, or find other ways to be preoccupied so they can avoid having to communicate with their roommates. They don't want to be alone, even though they may say they do, and they are often desperately lonely. They, too, lack the skills to express who they really are.

But the people-pleasers are lonely, too. We find a feeling of emptiness prevails among them, a fear that they're not enough or as much as they'd like to be.

One of the most important things we do is break that isolation by mandating contact with others. If patients consistently come back from their meetings and retire to their rooms to watch television, we will call them on their isolating behavior and tell them to start knocking on other people's doors. That simple act of taking the first step and the tentative "May I come in" is just as important as any insight they might have during a classroom lecture or therapy session, for they have taken an action and found out the real cause of their loneliness—themselves.

Another way we break the habit of isolation is by use of the buddy system. As soon as they enter treatment new patients are given a buddy who takes them around the unit, shows them where everything is, explains the schedule, and in the process enriches his or her own recovery by reaching out to help others. No matter where patients go for the twenty-eight days of treatment—for a walk, to the laundry, on a weekend pass—they go with a buddy. Lots of patients react intensely to the lack of privacy, but the truth is, being too private has allowed them to act self-destructively. We don't even let our patients cry in private. They've done too much of that already.

You can break out of the isolation you may be in at home by going to meetings of Overeaters Anonymous. There you will meet people who, like yourself, are willing to make profound changes to restore sanity in their lives. You may need more than an OA, however. You need a sponsor and you may need a therapist. Overeaters Anonymous is a support group, not a therapy group, and the meetings are really not a place to go to seek therapy.

Coping with an addiction in a group is a lot less painful than coping with it alone. I love the conference theme I used once: "We don't have it all together, but together we have it all." I have also noticed that people in 12-step meetings laugh a lot, not at jeering put-downs of others but at themselves. A room full of uproarious laughter is contagious and healing, and it takes the onus off recognizing you have an addiction. There are even those who come to see their addiction as a blessing, though it is not a requirement for membership in these wonderful fellowships. You can also break your isolation by reading this book with a buddy, with whom you are in constant contact. When you feel the need to reach out, your buddy will be there. When your buddy needs you, you'll be there, too. That kind of mutual support breeds self-respect.

GROUP THERAPY

In treatment, ground rules for therapy are: no gum chewing, smoking, or other distractions. Deal with the here and now, how you feel in the present moment. Speak for yourself in the first person, not of "you" or "we" but "I." Speak directly to an individual rather than to someone else about him or her. Be aware of the roles you play and your body messages. Be aware of how people in group remind you of other significant people in your life. Be an active listener. Expect periods of silence and postgroup feelings. A simple contract is made: to be honest, chemically free, and respect the confidentiality of the group. The same rules can apply to whatever group you choose to join during the twenty-eight days of this program, whether it is with a professional therapist or in an Anonymous meeting.

Ground rules for self-expression are very specific, for they clear the air of the smoke screen of nonfeelings and disbelief. Saying "I can't" is not allowed. It is a precondition of the mind, hardly ever of reality. It was once said that people can't go to the moon, can't fly, can't talk to each other over long distances through a wire, can't see pictures on a box in their living room. "Can't" is a self-limiting thought that means you haven't come up with the right combination of actions to make it happen. "I can't" is corrected to "I won't" at Janet Greeson's "A Place For Us."

"I don't know" is also not allowed. "I don't want to tell you" or "I don't believe in myself" or "I don't want to make the effort to find out" is what "I don't know" really means. "I'll try" is passive-aggressive. People don't change sitting on the fence. When that phrase is used at Janet Greeson's "A Place For Us" we say, "Trying is lying." "I should" is also forbidden, and anyone who uses it will be told to "Stop shoulding on yourself." The word "but" is also off limits. In a thought, it negates anything that comes before it.

Exaggerating is a device used to get people to be truthful about what they say and the way they say it. Anytime people say something in the victim mode, they're told to place the back of their hands dramatically on their foreheads. If they neglect to do so, others will provide the gesture for them.

At first it's frustrating to have so many restrictions put on the way you speak, but it eliminates the time-consuming, beating-around-the-bush babble that is allowed in more passive forms of therapy. There's no time for that in a 28-day program. Many patients who have been in long-term therapy, especially one-on-one, are often amazed to discover how much time and money they have wasted in self-indulgent verbalizing that never broke through their defenses to get to the heart of the matter—those explosive unexpressed feelings that lie behind layers of protective verbiage.

You can apply these ground rules for self-expression to your daily living, starting now. Be aware of how often you use the forbidden phrases. You will be amazed at how often others use them, too. Notice how they contribute to stuck thinking and cloudy communication. Try out your new way of expressing yourself in the safety of a 12-step meeting where honesty is encouraged and appreciated.

Within the small circle of eight to ten patients who meet with a counselor for group therapy four times a week, the most important work of treatment goes on, and the most intense bonding. People often come into treatment with no identity of their own. Once they get connected with a group, the other members help them see who they are and what they're doing. They first take on the identity of the group, and slowly out of that comes their own. People share things in a group they have told no one else in the world. Secrets, anger, grief, pain—much will be left behind in group during the twenty-eight days of treatment, and these are of greater significance than any weight lost or gained during that time.

As a therapist, I pretty much ignore people when they first come into group because I can be pretty intimidating. People are very nervous in the beginning because they think I know their secrets. Some I do know from my own experience, and they can feel that. In the beginning they're too nervous to be addressed, and if I do, I might push them farther back into themselves, so I just let them watch what's happening with patients who have been there longer. If new people do open up the first day or two, they rarely get to the real problem but put on a performance instead, full of defenses and devoid of real feeling. I'm more interested in getting them to relate to something someone else is saying.

I watch the eyes of patients for "tele"—the transmission of trust—when they are so closely bonded to the group that they are lost in what's happening in the moment. It's when they know I wouldn't let anything harmful happen to them, and they are willing to experience fully what they need to share. Achieving that trust is my goal as a group therapist. Not everybody is capable of that kind of vulnerability, but for those who are, miracles can happen.

HUGGING

Hugging can't be mandated, but it is an important part of treatment. Fat people generally don't get hugged a lot. Other people feel strange about hugging them, as if it were an intrusion. They sometimes perspire more than normal, they're not as sexually attractive as most people, and a lot of times are not sexually active either. Consequently, they develop touch deprivation or skin hunger, which they have learned to ignore.

I remember one time when denial of my skin hunger was broken through and nearly overwhelmed me. I was very overweight and hadn't been touched in a long time. I went to see the movie *Fatso* with a date who was extremely skinny. When he put his arm around me I almost died. I was flooded with feelings and realized how long it had been since I had been touched.

At first, some patients are uncomfortable with all the hugging that goes on, but they're so sensitive to touch they quickly become aware they're not touching people either, and that's part of recovery. People need to be hugged in a nonthreatening, nonsexual, nurturing way, and the contact fosters intimacy and trust much more rapidly than words. It's an amazing Rx—fast, simple, free, and nonfattening.

I'll never forget Terry, a bulimic who came into treatment looking like a little old lady, although she was in her early twenties. Every Monday we have commencement, a ceremony for the patients who are leaving treatment that week. Terry arrived that day. She wouldn't talk to anyone and kept her head down, appearing almost psychotic, as if she had lost touch with reality. At the close of the ceremony everyone stood in a circle and held hands. Someone tried to hug her and she angrily threw her arm away. After the ceremony, I went up to where she had withdrawn into a corner, put my hand on her arm, and said, "You're going to be okay. The only choice you have to make is whether your're going to let me help you," and she started crying.

Her twenty-eight days were rocky. Terry had been sexually abused by her father and had a very disapproving mother. She never felt comfortable at home, never felt as if she fit in anywhere, and was not even comfortable inside her own skin. During treatment, transference took place with me, and I became the loving support she never had, giving her lots of encouragement and support. Three years later, she's a vibrant, beautiful woman who's honest, positive, and so real she just throws off this incredible, wonderful energy. There's a real sense of joy in her heart, and she's full of hugs for everyone. She's a lover. You can be one, too.

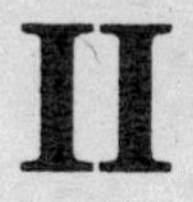

The Treatment Program

4

Week One

The Journey Begins

During the first week of treatment, as people go through withdrawal from drugs, alcohol, caffeine, sugar, work, outside relationships, or whatever they have been using to alter their mood, they are often too miserable to have the energy to keep up their usual defenses. We take advantage of the situation and do everything we can to penetrate their denial. No one wants to face being diagnosed as an addict, especially being addicted to a substance that is necessary to life! We break down the denial process in groups, identifying with each other to understand how isolation is the nature of the addiction. We also make patients aware of their defense mechanisms, which are the unique ways we protect who we think we are or hide who we think we're not. By the end of the first week, patients will have heard enough testimony about the nature of addiction to fully identify, and often discover it is not such a painful admission when it takes place in a group setting.

The second objective of the first week is to get people to identify and express their feelings. As you read this section, you will also be given many opportunities to identify yourself as a food addict, and tools in the workbook to help you get in touch with feelings and behavior you may have been working hard to deny.

Food Plan for the Next 28 Days

Prior to my own recovery, I was convinced that sugar was my only addictive substance. I went two years with the mentality "Lips that touch sugar will never touch mine," never recognizing that I was consuming three pounds of butter a week and the bread and potatoes to match.

I'm convinced food addiction is different for everyone. The key is "use" of food to negate, enhance, or stuff feelings. The food plan presented in the following pages is a guideline which will help you understand how you "use" food. Once you are aware of your patterns, you can change them.

Much research has been conducted at major medical centers during the past few years and their findings corroborate what I have believed in for a long time—that excessive calories are not the cause of obesity, fat intake is. It's not a sweet tooth that gives people problems so much as a fat tooth!

I recommend the following amounts for each of the plans outlined here:

Weight Loss Plan—15–20 percent fat
Weight Maintenance Plan—30–35 percent fat
Weight Gain Plan—45–50 percent fat

I recommend you limit your fat intake to 30 percent of the total calorie intake, at 9 calories per gram of fat. For instance, a 1,000-calorie limit would include 33 grams of fat. Although studies show that switching to a low-fat diet markedly increases the appetite for a few days, that ravenous period quickly passes. People who have lowered their fat intake in studies have not been found to compensate by eating more food.

Janet Greeson's "A Place For Us" Food Plan

Use the following food plan to help you plan your meals for the next 28 days. Be sure to consult with your physician in order to tailor the plan to meet your individual health needs.

WEIGHT LOSS PLAN

SAMPLE MENU

Breakfast

1 milk/dairy	4 oz. cottage cheese
1 fruit	1 medium apple
2 starches/grains	1 slice whole wheat toast
	½ cup corn bran
1 protein/meat	16 oz. skim milk
1 fat	1 teaspoon margarine for toast
	Decaf. coffee

Lunch

2 vegetables	1 cup raw salad (2 vegetables)
1 starch/grain	1 tablespoon low calorie dressing
1 protein/meat	4 oz. skinless chicken (baked or grilled)
	Water with lemon slice

Dinner

2 vegetables	1 cup mixed vegetables
1 starch/grain	½ cup brown rice
1 protein/meat	3 oz. lean beef
	Decaf. coffee

Nighttime Snack

1 fruit or	8 oz. plain yogurt
1 milk/dairy	
½ cup sugar-free gelatin	½ cup sugar-free gelatin

WEIGHT MAINTENANCE PLAN

SAMPLE MENU

Breakfast

1 milk/dairy	8 oz. skim milk
2 fruits	½ cup pineapple chunks
	½ cup unsweetened cinnamon applesauce
2 starches/grains	1 slice whole wheat toast
	½ cup oatmeal
1 protein/meat	1 tablespoon peanut butter
1 fat	(1 protein/meat and 1 fat)
	Herbal tea

Lunch

2 vegetables	½ cup sliced raw carrots
	½ broiled or raw medium tomato
2 starches/grains	2 slices whole wheat bread
2 proteins/meat	8 oz. tuna fish
1 fat	1 teaspoon mayonnaise
	Decaf. ice tea

Dinner

2 vegetables	1 cup raw salad
1 fruit	½ cup unsweetened mandarin oranges and sliced bananas
2 starches/grains	1 medium baked sweet potato
	½ cup cooked peas
1 protein/meat	3 oz. grilled pork chop
1 fat	1 tablespoon low calorie dressing
1 milk/dairy	8 oz. skim milk
	Decaf. coffee

Nighttime Snack

1 fruit or	½ cup cantaloupe
1 milk/dairy	
½ cup sugar-free gelatin	½ cup sugar-free gelatin

WEIGHT GAIN PLAN

SAMPLE MENU

Breakfast

1 milk/dairy	8 oz. plain yogurt
2 fruits	½ small banana
	½ grapefruit
2 starches/grains	½ cup of puffed rice
	1 slice of wheat toast
1 protein/meat	16 oz. skim milk
1 fat	1 teaspoon margarine
	Decaf. coffee

Lunch

2 vegetables	1 cup raw cauliflower and carrots
2 fruits	4 tablespoons of raisins
3 starches/grains	2 slices of wheat bread
	2 rice cakes
2 proteins/meat	6 oz. lean roast beef
1 fat	1 teaspoon mayonnaise
	Decaf. sugar-free soda

Dinner

2 starches/grains	1 medium baked potato
	1 medium ear of corn
2 vegetables	1 cup steamed broccoli pieces
2 fats	4 oz. grated low-fat mozzarella cheese
1 protein/meat	4 oz. baked fish
2 fruits	¾ cup sliced strawberries
	½ cup sliced honeydew melon
1 milk/dairy	½ cup low-fat cottage cheese
	Herbal tea

Nighttime Snack

1 fruit or	1 medium apple
1 milk/dairy	
½ cup sugar-free gelatin	½ cup sugar-free gelatin

Recommended Food List and Portion Sizes

PROTEIN

Meats

Red meat (lean beef, veal, lean pork, lamb)—3 ounces
Poultry (chicken, turkey, goose, capon, Cornish hen) Remove skin before eating—4 ounces
Fish and shellfish—4 ounces (Canned fish should be packed in water)

Dairy or nonmeat proteins

Eggs—2 medium
Dried beans, cooked—1 cup
Cottage cheese—4 ounces or ½ cup
Hard cheese—2 ounces
Low-fat plain yogurt—1 cup or 8 ounces
Tofu—4 ounces
Milk (skim or nonfat)—8 ounces—1 dairy or ½ protein portion
Skim buttermilk—8 ounces—1 dairy or ½ protein portion
Peanut butter (unsweetened)—1 tablespoon (add 1 fat)

VEGETABLES

½ cup

Alfalfa sprouts
Artichoke
Asparagus
Bamboo shoots
Bean sprouts
Beans—yellow and green
Beets
Bok choy
Broccoli
Brussel sprouts
Cabbage
Carrots
Cauliflower
Celery
Chard
Chicory
Chinese cabbage
Collards
Cucumber
Dandelion greens
Eggplant
Endive
Escarole
Jicama
Kale
Lettuce
Mushrooms
Mustard greens
Okra
Onions
Parsley
Pepper, green/red

Pickles, dill
Pimientos
Radishes
Raw salad
Rhubarb
Rutabagas
Sauerkraut
Snow pea pods
Spinach
Sprouts
Squash (zucchini, summer, winter, yellow, spaghetti, etc.)
String beans
Tomatoes
Tomato juice, V-8
4 oz. = 1 portion
Turnips
Watercress
Water chestnuts

FRUITS

Apple—1 medium
Apple juice—½ cup
Applesauce (sugar-free)—½ cup
Apricots (unsweetened)—3 medium
Banana—½ small
Berries—½ cup
Cantaloupe—½ cup
Casaba, cranshaw—¼ melon
Cranberry juice (sugar-free)—1 cup
Fruit cocktail (sugar-free)—1 cup, not including the juice
Grapefruit—½
Honeydew—¼ melon
Lemons/limes—2
Nectarines—2 small or 1 large
Orange—1 medium/juice—1 cup
Peach—1
Pineapple—1 cup or ¼ pineapple
Plums—2
Prune juice—½ cup
Raisins (unsweetened)—2 tablespoons
Rhubarb—1 cup
Strawberries—¾ cup
Tangerines—2
Watermelon—1 cup

Avoid exotic fruits.

Juice is a poor substitute for fresh fruit and we suggest

that you use it only when fresh fruit is unavailable. Buy fruit that is canned in juice, not corn syrup. Drain juice before eating.

STARCHES/GRAINS

½ cup unless stated otherwise

Barley, cooked
Beans—lima, navy, etc.
Bread—no white flour
Buckwheat
Corn (no sugar)
  kernels—½ cup
  ear—1 medium
Corn bran
Grape-Nuts—no sugar
Grits, cooked
Groats, cooked
Kidney beans, cooked
Oat bran, cooked—4 teaspoons
Oatmeal, cooked
Parsnips—⅔ cup
Peas—dried (cooked)
Potato—baked—1 medium
  mashed—½ cup
  Sweet—1 small
Pumpkin—¾ cup
Rice—brown, puffed, 2 rice cakes
Shredded wheat
Wheat bran
Wheat germ—¼ cup
Yams

OILS, FATS

one teaspoon unless otherwise indicated

Butter—be aware that it is an animal fat, which is high in cholesterol
Corn oil
Margarine (polyunsaturated only)
Olive oil

Safflower oil
Salad dressing—(one tablespoon)—sugar must be the 5th listed ingredient or lower
Sunflower oil
Vegetable oil

CONDIMENTS

—No more than 1 teaspoon per day of spices
—No more than 1 ounce per day of sauces

Bouillon (fat free, low salt)
Cinnamon
Extracts (imitation, alcohol-free, such as vanilla)
Ketchup (sugar-free)
Lemon juice
Mayonnaise (low calorie)
Mustard
Salsa
Salt substitute
Soy sauce (light, low salt)
Spices and seasonings (sugar-free)
Tamari sauce (low salt)
Vinegar
Worcestershire sauce

THESE ITEMS NEED TO BE AVOIDED AT ALL TIMES

Alcohol
Caffeine (coffee, tea, chocolate, soda, etc.)
Corn starch
Corn sweetener
Fried foods
Honey
Pasta containing white flour
Pizza made with white flour
Salt
Snack foods, including chips, pretzels, nuts
Sugar (dextrose, fructose, lactose, sucrose, glucose, white flour)

Any foods that can trigger a binge should be avoided.

Day One
DEFENSE MECHANISMS

Our minds may deceive us but our bodies never lie. The autonomic nervous system has a life of its own and pays no attention to what the mind wants to project to the outside world. When it feels like blushing, it blushes. When it feels like crying, it cries. When it's alarmed, it breaks out in gooseflesh. Because of this truth-telling disparity between mind and body, when people first come to Janet Greeson's "A Place For Us" we watch as much as we listen. Their actions speak so loudly we can hardly hear a word they're saying, and we know that no matter what they try to convey to us with words, their nonverbal language tells the truth.

Some are full of shame. Their eyes are cast down, they readily weep, they cover their face with their hands when they talk as if they had something to hide, they are angry at themselves and feel empty or numb. The very obese are often suicidally depressed. Nothing seems to work for them now, and they have completely submerged their identity under layers of fat. The heaviest patient I had weighed 470 pounds. She was barely able to get herself dressed and thought she had no reason for living except to eat herself to death.

Most people come in depressed. Some are hostile, blaming others for their problems, angry at everyone but themselves and full of complaints. Gerald G. Jampolsky, MD, author of *Teach Only Love,* remarks, "The most offensive patients are the ones who need the most love." Sometimes that's difficult to remember, but I've never failed to acknowledge the truth of that statement.

Still other people are placid. They will calmly tell you there's nothing the matter with them except a need to control their weight. They will go out of their way to please people and do whatever they can to get approval.

Surprisingly, the passive people are the most difficult to treat, for there is no struggle. The shame-based people are struggling with themselves, the anger-based people are struggling against the world, but the passive people-pleasers are not struggling against anything. They want somebody to fix them without taking action themselves.

In order to get the passive types to work, we have to shake them up a bit. We don't respond to their need to please. Getting them to drop their defensive behavior is no game; if we can't shake them out of their passivity, they usually go home without doing any real work on their emotions and don't get better. What I do is make them into bad patients. I'm always glad when I see their anger and feistiness begin to come out. My nurses say they don't like them as well as they did when they first came on the unit, but that's okay by me. They're learning to challenge and create boundaries, developing an identity beyond just being nice.

People who are full of guilt and shame often don't know why, or give erroneous reasons for the way they feel. In their intake interview they may deny or claim they are not aware of anything in their childhood that caused them to feel so bad about themselves, but the red flag is up to look for abuse. These people are often the ones who go right to work. As soon as they begin to respond to a safe and loving environment, they are so needy and grateful they begin to express their pain.

Passive people, on the other hand, are so numb their deep-seated pain needs time to surface, and much is done during treatment to stimulate it to rise. In the words of the psychotherapist Dr. Elvin Semrod, "When you feel nothing, *that's* when you hurt the most."

Before angry people can get down to work, they must struggle through their denial. They may refuse to admit that they are the problem or even that they have one, but once they do, the energy is there to work with. When I was counseling in Navy alcohol treatment centers, I found the people who were referred against their will actually did better than the ones who came into treatment voluntarily. The recalcitrant ones were constantly telling me, "Screw you, I'm no alkie," while the people who came into treatment on their own weren't struggling with their denial at all.

There is often a secondary denial that lies beneath the surface of an open admission of addiction. Sometimes this denial emerges when a person returns home after treatment when it might lead to a relapse. I often wonder if people openly in denial get a lot more attention by therapists during treatment, and consequently they may avoid having to go through the anguish of secondary denial.

KINDS OF DEFENSES

The behaviors people use as defense mechanisms keep the world at arm's length and their true feelings buried. *Blaming* is a form of protection. People who play the victim role are often rigid in their belief that the world is out to get them, and they are never the reason for their problems. I like to tell people that every time I point a finger at you there are three fingers pointing back at me. I recognize a fault in you because I have it in me, and that makes me mad! *Judging* is a related form of defense. Those who are the harshest judges of others are also the hardest on themselves, and this provides a clue to work with them on elevating their self-esteem.

Patronizing is a favorite defense of those who feel inferior to others. They project a false sense of superiority for protection. Patronizing is especially common among patients who hold some status in the outside world. They wear their arrogance as a mask until they feel safe enough to discard it. Others use *intellectualizing*, *explaining*, and *justifying*, doing a lot of verbal gymnastics to avoid identifying their feelings. They are often skilled at another defense, *generalizing*.

Projecting is another common defense mechanism. People who use it will confront others for something they do themselves. Whenever a patient becomes upset over the behavior of another patient in treatment, it usually means they are observing what they don't like about themselves.

Smiling and complying are defenses used a lot by people-pleasers. *Withdrawing* or going into a deep *depression* are defenses used by passive types who work hard at making people guess what's wrong with them. They may get annoyed when I tell them, "I'm not a good guesser. You'll have to *tell* me what's wrong." I am a good guesser, because I know how to read nonverbal behavior, but I won't play into their defenses. Then there are those who use *joking* or *minimizing* as a defense.

People can use any of these defense mechanisms occasionally and the behavior may be seen as a protective reaction to a particularly stressful situation, not a habitual practice. We look for patterns, behaviors people use consistently. None of these mechanisms work in treatment. They are identified for what they are—behaviors that mask true feelings—first by the counselors and then by the others in treatment.

People develop defense mechanisms to protect themselves when they lack other resources. There's always a payoff and we have to help them figure out what the payoff is. When it's identified, people often recoil with distaste at finding they exhibit the very behavior they abhor in others, and they work hard to find a more truthful way to present themselves.

Workbook for Day One

ASSIGNMENT ONE: RECOGNIZING DEFENSE MECHANISMS YOU USE

This is difficult to do by yourself because you have worked hard building your defense system, and you are as reluctant to consider the need for it. You have invested a lot in your defenses, and you are not going to give them up willingly! I have constructed situations to which hypothetical people respond, using the kinds of defense mechanisms discussed in today's classroom, giving first a sample response, and then the payoff. Make an honest search of your own behavior, and if you identify any of the mechanisms as ones you use, put a check mark by it. Next week you will be asked to review the list again, and hopefully you will be willing then to see what you resist identifying with now.

______Blaming

Johanna failed to pass her licensing exam: "The test was biased. I was distracted because my daughter had smashed the fender of my car. I was coming down with a cold, and the instructor who prepared me for the exam emphasized all the wrong things. No wonder I failed."

Payoff: Johanna doesn't have to face the fact that she didn't study hard enough.

______Projecting

Ralph's son has trouble making friends. "He doesn't seem to realize that his attitude leaves a lot to be desired. I tried to teach him how to make friends, but he won't listen. He's stuck-up and is always complaining. I can't imagine how he got that way. I have always been a good influence."

Payoff: By projecting onto his son the very character defects he has, and that his son has learned from him, Ralph doesn't have to examine his own behavior.

______Judging

Mona's neighbor's teenage children are in trouble with the law again. She tells another neighbor, "If their mother had stayed at home with those children when they were growing up, they wouldn't be in trouble like this now."

Payoff: Mona feels a sense of moral superiority making this judgment. It also corroborates her own decision to forsake a career to stay home with *her* children when they were growing up, which she now feels too insecure to pursue.

______Patronizing

Jim's fiancée is studying to be a lawyer: "She's becoming quite the little grind, just buries that cute nose of hers in the books for days at a time. I tell her at this rate she'll be a better lawyer than I am."

Payoff: By diminishing his fiancée's efforts, Jim increases his status and minimizes the possible threat of career conflict.

______Explaining

Maria has an argument with her sister: "I haven't been able to get along with her for years. When we were little, she used to pick on me and she's never stopped. Dad always preferred her, and Mom took my side, so there was never any possibility for us to work out things between ourselves. My sister lives in the past and can't see Dad no longer respects her, because she's just not aware situations change. I think that's because when she was a little kid she was sick a lot and got shut down. She lives in a dream world."

Payoff: By minutely examining the psychological motives of her sister, Maria can avoid looking at the real reason for the conflict.

_____Intellectualizing

Rose is lonely: "My inability to make friends stems from a childhood spent with adults who enriched my life greatly, took me to cultural events, read me great literature, and heightened my awareness far beyond the normal capacity of a child. To this day I need to be overstimulated. Only a well-read, well-developed mind is able to keep my interest. I would rather stay home and read great literature than spend time at a party where people talk of trivial things. I put a high value on my mental capacity and am willing to forsake the friendship of others if they can't appreciate it."

Payoff: Rose can avoid the risk of being with people who might surpass her mental capacity. She can stay at home and continue to believe that she is the brightest one she knows.

_____Generalizing

Al didn't get into the college of his choice: "They never take people from my part of the country. They always want to fill up their enrollment with students from the East or West Coast. I also heard too many people who want to study engineering applied this year. Or maybe it's just they don't like people of my ethnic persuasion."

Payoff: Al cushions his disappointment by making blanket statements about why he was rejected, thus avoiding having to take it personally.

_____People-Pleasing

Sandra is running for president of her block association: "I have a hundred phone calls to make today. I'm baking a little something for my next-door neighbor, who's under the weather, and need to drop in on my sister-in-law. She could stand for some cheering up after her accident. Then I told the outgoing president of our group that I'd take care of the mailing, so I have to get to the post office. Two people said they'd help and they've both canceled. I guess I'll just do it myself. It will save time in the end."

Payoff: By busily doing everyone favors, Sandra can feel important. She can also mask the fact that no one ever does her any favors, so busy doing instead of being.

______Withdrawing

Patrick has asked a woman friend to go to a dinner dance and has been turned down: "I really didn't want to go anyway. I hate those affairs. I can put the time to good use by finishing a report this weekend and cleaning the garage. I like being by myself. I'm good company and always spend my time alone productively. Dances and social affairs always end up making me feel like I'm wasting time and money."

Payoff: By not asking someone else, he avoids the pain of further rejection.

______Depression

Judith didn't get picked for the vocal competition: "What's the use? I work and work and someone else comes along who doesn't even study voice and gets it. Nothing comes easy for me. Why is it always like that? I've been disappointed so many times I don't know why I continue to torture myself. The hell with it. I'm through trying to get anywhere. I'm just wasting my time."

Payoff: Judith's defeated attitude protects her from trying further. Feeling sorry for herself is at least some comfort, and the bad mood she's in keeps others away, confirming her worst fears about herself.

______Joking

Mary Lou has to buy a new swimsuit because last year's is too small: "Oh, look, a sale on cabana wear. Why don't I just buy the cabana? Remember the tent dress? I might start a new fashion trend."

Payoff: Her friends laugh and Mary Lou hides her shame at having put on so much weight.

______Minimizing

Rosalie got turned down for an appointment she badly wanted: "Oh, it's nothing. I wasn't ready to make any changes anyway. It's not that much of a promotion and the salary differential is peanuts because it would have put me in a new tax bracket. Besides, it's up on a different floor and I would have had to make all new friends."

Payoff: She saves face with her coworkers and doesn't have to acknowledge her disappointment.

If you checked off less than three defense mechanisms, you have some soul-searching to do. If you checked off six or more, you're working hard. If you checked off more than ten, you might be being a little hard on yourself.

ASSIGNMENT TWO: AFFIRMATION—YOU ARE A CELEBRATION OF LIFE!

Affirmations are messages to your own inner healing nature, the part of you that wants to grow, change, and be joyful. They need to be said many times for them to take root and grow in your unconscious where they can begin to effect change. You will feel the change first when you are less than fully conscious, particularly when you wake up in the morning. You will be aware that you are less anxious, more peaceful, more willing to change. I can't explain how this happens, only that it does.

If you are troubled by the use of the word "God" in an affirmation, substitute for it in your mind a word that does not trouble you, or think of it as standing for "good orderly direction." It's just a word, but the concept of a beneficial power in the universe greater than your own is important to making this program work. I have come to believe there *is* a God—in us all, and all around us. It is the power of love and the joy of beauty, and it can't be used against you or anyone.

This is a very short affirmation from *The Course of Miracles.* You may easily memorize it. Say it aloud to yourself as many times as you remember during the day, especially before going to sleep:

I am not my body
I am free
I am as God created me.

ASSIGNMENT THREE: DIARY

Beginning today, keep a diary, not of your activities but of your thoughts, feelings, frustrations—what you say, learn, and come to understand—while working through the twenty-eight days. Make each entry as long or as short as you need, but write something every day. In this way you can measure your own progress and can make written commitments to yourself that are directed toward self-improvement. This diary will serve to strengthen your program of abstinence and recovery.

In order for this diary to serve any useful purpose in your life, it must be completed honestly and fearlessly. The entries are made by you, about you, and for you, and need to be shown to no one.

The act of writing helps us to formulate and clarify our thoughts, feelings, and observations. If you really work this program, you are going to experience many changes, and you need to write them down to process them. Writing also helps us to commit ourselves to our own conscious unfolding. We are taking a step beyond simply thinking something when we make the effort to write it down. The more frequently we write, the easier it becomes until one day you sit down and the words begin to flow out of the pen. Then what you write becomes really valuable to your understanding, releasing the contents of your heart into your fingers, bypassing your head.

Because we cannot write down all our thoughts, we must choose the ones that are most important. In the process, we get more in touch with our sense of values.

Writing is also a great stimulus to creativity. In writing down our conscious thoughts, useful associations and new ideas begin to emerge. Writing the immediate thoughts makes more "room" for new avenues of thinking, new possibilities we may not have considered before.

As a psychological journal, it can also serve as a harmless and effective technique of expressing feelings by giving us the opportunity to write about whatever powerful or disruptive emotion we may have bottled up inside us. The process of "letting off steam" through writing is one that many have found extremely productive, for not only does it discharge tension, it also enables us to become aware of some of the underlying issues behind such tensions.

Drawings and other visual material can also be an important part of your journal. These may be images that come in the form of dreams, fantasies, or visualizations. Recording your dreams will increase your recall. You may want to keep your journal by your bedside so you can write them down immediately upon waking while they are still fresh in your mind. The images evoked in dreams are often early clues to new changes and revelations about to occur in your conscious mind. The more you record them, the more access you will have to your dream life. Spontaneous drawings are also highly useful. These are made by putting pen to paper without any preconceived idea of what they will be like. The result can be of considerable value in self-understanding.

This diary is not a mere recording of facts, such as what you did with whom, or what you had for lunch. It is about feelings, particularly strong feelings, peak experiences, any "high" or "deep" feelings of peace, joy, love, expansion, awakening, their circumstances and effects. Also include the negative feelings you have, and remember that strong negative reactions you have to other people may clarify your own unrecognized and projected problems.

Also record the techniques for change you are consciously using, and other unplanned experiences or situations that you find helpful in your ongoing growth process. This diary is also to be used as an honest recording of your personal weaknesses, character defects, and limitations that you want to be more aware of so you can work to change them. But give particular emphasis to the positive by including your successes—instances in which you did use the new tools you are learning to overcome the limitations. Include bright ideas that come to you, fantasies, stories, and situations that have special meaning to you and that may serve as seeds for further imaginative work. Record quotations you may have read or heard that are personally meaningful to you.

Use dialogue in your journal entries. We often find ourselves carrying on an imaginary conversation with a person, or rehearsing an important event. Used consciously and deliberately, the inner dialogue can help us clarify our relationships to specific people, developing understanding and evoking insight. It is also possible to have a dialogue with things other than persons, for instance with ideas and events. We can have a dialogue with the idea itself, or with a figure we construct that embodies the idea.

Writing down internal dialogues that many of us engage in is also helpful. When we write out the dialogue rather than merely imagine it, we can reread it and study its content and meaning. One of the characteristics of these imaginary dialogues is they are more monologues than conversations. When we write down what we imagine the other person will say, his or her point of view may become clearer to us, and underlying motivations may reveal themselves to an extent that would not be possible in an unmonitored imaginary dialogue.

There is another form of dialogue that is helpful to write down, a simple and straightforward conversation with your own higher self. Within each of us is an endowment of wisdom, intuition, and a sense of purpose that can become a source of guidance in everyday life once we acknowledge its presence and validate its opinion. Trust the assumption that it is there and it will answer you.

A final word: Trust the process of keeping a daily diary. It is a bridge from where you were to where you are and where you hope to be.

A Day in the Life
ELAINE

Day one. First moment since I got up this morning that I've had time to write in this diary we're supposed to keep. Last night when I came in, there was a sign right off the elevator: "Welcome to Janet Greeson's 'A Place For Us' with three names: Elaine, Tony, Jean. Made me feel good to know I'm not the only new kid in town. This place is pleasant, and not at all institutional. There are pretty pictures and prints on the wall. Nice, like it says we're worth something.

Two people hugged me, which made me feel taken aback. One said, "You're scared now, but you'll be all right." I wasn't scared, just numb. My roommate was banging around for what seemed like hours. She's a real angry person. I tried to talk to her and she just completely ignored me.

It was still dark this morning when I woke up. Suddenly I felt a wave of depression come over me, like there's an insurmountable task before me and I'm not up to it. I don't know how I will ever manage to stay here for twenty-eight days.

Breakfast was at seven o'clock, the earliest I've eaten in years. Eating an egg without toast was very depressing. The decaf coffee was a bummer. I could really use a jolt of caffeine. Sat next to a real heavy, sweet guy named Mike who talked a lot. He said after a few days of caffeine withdrawal I'd feel even worse. I told him thanks a lot. Also talked to a woman who says she's lost seventeen pounds since she came three weeks ago. "But that's not as important as what else I lost—a lot of garbage in my head, a lot of grief." People who have been here for a while (my roommate Gloria being the exception) are pretty caring. That makes me feel less anxious. The dining room reminds me of high school. I'm having a hard time learning the names of twenty-four people all at once.

Smitty did my intake interview. He kept asking me if there were problems with my childhood. I told him I was fortunate to have good parents. My father died so many years ago I hardly ever think about him, and I'm not exactly on good terms with Mom because she's so difficult, but I have nothing to complain about compared to some of the people here like the poor woman I went walking with this morning, Linda, just skin and bones. I felt so huge next to her.

People come into treatment and leave at different times, so Monday the ones who are leaving this week graduated in a nice little ceremony upstairs. There were six of them, all smiles. The counselors gave them little plaques and talked about how they had changed. One thing I've noticed, when the counselors introduce themselves, they say they're recovering addicts of one kind or another. There's lots of joking around here about being addicts. I'm not at all comfortable with that.

At the close of graduation we all stood in a circle and sang. People cried. I did, too. I don't know why, just because the others did I guess. There's so many sad cases here I really feel for them.

There's a coffee machine in a little kitchenette across from my room. I'm in there constantly, hoping to get a kick. The cups are too small. Lunch was pretty good: cold cuts and cheese, fruit cup. More decaf. I miss bread. Linda the anorexic was sitting alone and I joined her. There was so much food on her plate—stewed beef over brown rice, stewed tomatoes, custard, plus bread and butter! I really don't think it's fair that we all eat together. I was secretly angry at her when she said she hated to waste food and this was much more than she could possibly eat. I wanted to reach over and wolf down that stew with my bare hands. She asked if I'd like some of her food and I reminded her we weren't supposed to do that. Went and had some more decaf to calm down.

2:30. Just came out of my first group therapy. It was very scary. I'm a jumble of nerves from it. Have to write it down before I block it out. A woman read a letter to her mother's boyfriend, who had sexually abused her. It got pretty graphic. Her hands were shaking so bad she couldn't hold the letter. Smitty put a chair in front of her with a regular bed pillow in it. She was crying and raging away. He had someone else hold the chair down. She was beating the pillow so hard with her fists the chair was moving. Smitty kept telling her to use her open palm. "You've hurt yourself enough for what he did." He sat right by her, talking to her calmly as if everything were as normal as can be. I was absolutely terrified. They will never get me to do this. I hope it's not required. She raged and raged and said the most awful things, and then when she started coming out of it, Smitty said was there more and she said, "Yes!" and then started in about her mother: "You knew! And you did nothing about it!" If I could have gotten out of there, I would have. Afterward Smitty asked her if there was someone in the group who could comfort her, and she went and sat on this woman Mary's lap like a little child. Mary kept stroking her hair and telling her she was going to be all right. Smitty asked the others in group to talk to her. Tony, a big blustery Italian, looked like he wanted to cry and told her she was brave. I wanted to say something but the words wouldn't come out. Smitty said to me, "What's going on for you, Elaine?" and I said, "Nothing." He told me I didn't have to smile so much. That made me angry but I didn't say anything.

5 P.M. Dinner is so early! I'd finished eating by five-fifteen. The thought that I'd not get anything to eat until seven the next morning threw me into a panic. "Don't worry," someone said, "we get a piece of fruit before we go to bed." A piece of fruit? I don't know how I'm going to stand this. I'm so depressed. I want to go home. I hate group therapy, all that spilling your guts out.

6:30 P.M. We got bused to an Overeaters Anonymous meeting in a church about twenty minutes away. It was great! One woman got up and talked about how she had been lying to her group back home for the past eight months and stopped going because of it. She started to cry and couldn't finish. By the time the meeting was over she was laughing. Everyone was so supportive, congratulating me on my first day of abstinence. I really liked the attitude of the people there. It didn't seem to matter whether you ate too much or too little. The thing was how you felt about yourself and that was invariably the same—lousy! All the way home I kept thinking about that piece of fruit, spent a lot of time deciding between the apple and the pear. Practically ate it core and all.

Midnight. Can't get to sleep. Keep thinking of what happened in group with the woman who beat the chair with the pillow. All that rage! Where did it come from?

Day Two
VALUES, ATTITUDES, AND BELIEFS

You may be wondering how people can turn their lives around in twenty-eight days, especially when they may have spent a lifetime trying unsuccessfully to do just that! The answer is, you can't turn a life around unless you find a direction it's preferable to go in. Nature abhors a vacuum; one belief can't be removed without substituting it with another. In treatment we systematically replace destructive, negative thought and behavior with loving behavior—that is, such that will be constructive, productive, and additive in your life, increase your self-esteem and your self-worth.

How long you have held food as a value can help us make the distinction as to who needs treatment. There is a timetable for behavior change, depending upon the duration of the behavior that needs to be changed. A *value,* something you hold for what it is, or for its own sake, is developed one to five years in length of the experience. To change a value will take ten to fifteen hours of instruction and equal commitment.

An *attitude* is a viewpoint that you have had that you really need your substance of choice to exist. It involves your physical, mental, emotional, and spiritual habits, and it is difficult to change. It is the value you hold for food plus time, between five to ten years in length of the experience. To change an attitude will take twenty to thirty-six hours of instruction and equal commitment.

A *belief* is a strongly held commitment developed over time through the integration of values and attitudes. If you've held food as an important integral part of your life for more than ten years, or have been using food to cope with life for more than ten years, your belief will require at least thirty days to change. You have spent a long time in a relationship with food instead of people and need to change some deeply held convictions about yourself. You will be working through this section of the book on faith. I commend you for that and encourage you to keep slogging on even when you are convinced you will fail. Remember the timetable. It can't be shortened but it *does work.*

If you have always isolated yourself from your feelings, you probably have a big problem trusting others and believe you are basically unlovable. That deeply help belief is particularly difficult to change, impossible without a loving and nurturing environment. But it can be changed, and frequently is at Janet Greeson's "A Place For Us." When people come into treatment who don't know how to be a social being, we teach them how. We love them until they can love themselves. This kind of change takes place not just with the help of the staff but with the others in treatment, for they quickly learn that healing takes place when they give to others, and that giving back is what nudges out the old behavior. Often the people who come in the most shut down are the ones who become the most responsive to the loneliness and awkward feelings of the newcomer. In a span of two or three weeks they are giving back in full measure the gift they have just received.

The process of behavior change is one of DO, FEEL, and BELIEVE. You can think until you disappear into your navel. You've got to *act*. Think of all the self-help books you have read that had only momentary effect on your life. That's because your participation was passive. **"You can't think your way into good action but you can act your way into good thinking."** The best way to increase your self-esteem is to do "esteemable" things!

Behavior precedes feeling: you don't hurt until you stub your toe. If you take an action, even if you don't understand why you're doing it and have no idea what's going to happen, afterward you will feel something—either better or worse. As a result of that feeling your attitude will shift one way or another, and after enough shift in attitude, your belief will follow.

In the twenty-eight days of treatment, you will be doing a lot of things that you don't understand, until one day you feel a change in the way you feel. At that point, you won't need to examine why these actions work or even how they work, for you'll know they do work. Food addiction is a disease about feelings. Because they're part of the problem, they're also part of the solution. They are the way in and the way out. You will know you are working this program when you feel it working in you.

Workbook for Day Two

ASSIGNMENT ONE: VALUE, ATTITUDE, BELIEF CLARIFICATION CHART

Divide a sheet of paper into three columns and label the columns "Value," "Attitude," and "Belief." The first column will be for things, people, and activities—whatever you have put a value on for less than five years. The second column is for things you have valued for the past five to ten years, and the third for things you have valued for longer than ten years.

For example, let's say you chose three things you have valued for less than five years: 1. motorcycle riding, 2. Saturday dinners with the neighbors, and 3. working for yourself. For each, describe whether you: 1. do it alone or with others, 2. whether your mother and/or father valued it, 3. whether you want people you love to value it, 4. whether eating is involved, and 5. the last time you did it.

By the time your chart is finished, you will get a good clarification of what kinds of value you give things in your life, and whether you are consistent or changing in what you value. Consider the values you now have and think ahead to five years from now. Would you like them to be the same or different in the future? If the same, how can you enrich them further? If different, how can they be replaced with something better?

ASSIGNMENT TWO: CHANGING VALUES

What changes would you like to make—in your values, your attitudes, your beliefs, your lifestyle—whatever you see going on in your life that is keeping you from being happy? Make a list.

ASSIGNMENT THREE: YOU ARE A CELEBRATION OF LIFE!

Affirmation: Imagine Who You Are and Then Create Yourself.

What qualities do you want to possess in greater measure?

You are now going to compose a personalized affirmation to add to the short affirmation you memorized yesterday. Your personalized affirmation is made up of the statement "I am" followed by the qualities you listed above, and incorporating the changes you want to make. Remember, an affirmation is positive self-talk, what you say to yourself under your breath, by which you can replace those destructive negative messages you may be muttering to yourself all the time. Think of them as a cassette tape and your new messages as erasing the old.

For example, let's say you listed among the changes a desire to (1) lose forty pounds, (2) change professions, and (3) develop a better relationship with significant people in your life. In the qualities you want to possess you listed (1) self-confidence, (2) attractiveness, (3) success, and (4) serenity. To make your personal affirmation, you write:

"I am lovable. I am flexible and full of courage. I am fun to be with, and I care about others. I am attractive, successful, and serene. I am capable of achieving whatever goal I set for myself."

Don't wince. You *are* capable of being all these things, and putting them in the present tense will make them happen. Your real self is yearning for this information and will readily begin to act on it, but that internal healer in you is also very literal. If you give it a command in the future tense, it will put off acting until the future. If you affirm that you are now what you want to become, it will begin at once to work for you. Remember "do, feel, believe." You won't feel and you won't believe until you do. Doing without belief is called faith. It *does* move mountains—by giving you a shovel and the will to do the job.

Make copies of this personalized affirmation and

tape it to your refrigerator, post it above your desk, keep it at your bedside, and repeat it throughout the day, every day, throughout the week, until you begin to feel the results.

A Day in the Life
JEAN

Day two, 7:30 A.M. As I brushed my teeth, I heard an old Iggy Pop song in my head: "Don't no one try to tell me what to do." I feel so rebellious. I fear losing my identity. This hospital armband bothers me. Things I don't like: rules. Too many restrictions. The rule bothering me the most is #26: "No patients are to use the stairs at the end of the hall by room 217 or 201. No patients are to be on roof or throw anything out of window." It's sinister. It makes me want to go on the stairs. What would anyone throw out a window? An SOS? "Send chocolate?"

After breakfast I feel better. Everyone here seems in good spirits today. They are all different ages, from different parts of the country, and vastly different sizes. There's a big, gentle man, Mike, and a nineteen-year-old wiseguy named Tim who said he dreamed about crack. He scoffed, "If I shared that in group, someone will say, 'Oh, I can relate, I dreamed I ate a Hostess cupcake.'" Obviously he doesn't see food addiction as being as serious as drug addiction. I wonder why he's here.

11 A.M. Walk. I feel the sun go right through my head. It hurts. We're supposed to try to go around the fitness course three times, but I only make it once, very slowly.

6 P.M. This is free time and I appreciate it. Blanche, my therapist in group, says my buddy Debbie and I are a lot alike. We're smiling depressives and we need to cry more. I seem to be crying a lot and I don't like it. I have a visual miasma from the withdrawal of everything—caffeine, sugar, alcohol. Blanche says I don't have to get involved with other people's problems, but it's hard because their stories are so sad—incest, battering, extreme obesity, and painful thinness.

This hospital makes me feel like a child, so I might as well be a child. I'm supposed to be just in a feeling state;

if I'm sad, my face can show it. I tried it out on the psychological tester and found it hard not to match her smile because I thought I'd hurt her feelings, but I got over it. It felt powerful, like I have the beginnings of integrity.

Blanche also said I don't trust people because my parents couldn't be trusted. This is true. I have been so tough and strong all these years because I didn't know what else to do. Now that I'm here and there's nothing to do, I feel powerless. That's supposed to be the first step of OA, but it feels like nowhere. Perhaps acknowledged nowhere is more real than whatever there was before. A fake life? It didn't feel that way, but there were plenty of lies.

10 P.M. They gave me Decamethazol, a pill that will test for chemical depression. It interacts with cortisone in the system. They said there are no side effects. I have a pile of program literature and endless questionnaires to fill out before curfew. Curfew? I feel like I'm in a war novel.

Day Three
SOCIAL SKILLS

Today I want you to feel as if you're back in kindergarten, because we are going to be discussing the most elementary matter: social skills—what children are taught when they first go to school and interact with their peers. If you balk at having to focus on such simple matters, may I remind you once again that addiction is a disease of isolation. Focusing on social skills is as appropriate to treating addiction as aspirin is to treating a fever.

Sometimes social skills were never learned, or forgotten. Lack of social skills is magnified in adolescence, when the onset of sexuality makes life even more complicated. Hardly anyone gets through that difficult phase of life unscathed, and many of us still feel like adolescents when we enter a room full of strangers at a party, or wait for our first dinner guests to arrive.

Why should it be so hard to be a social being? I say, it's not. In fact, it's so easy it's laughable! To be at ease, all you have to do is put others at ease, look them in the eye, listen to what they say, tell them what's on your mind, and lo and behold—a conversation! Add to that a little laughter, a few hugs, and you've got social skills.

NAMES

You meet someone new and are introduced. Did you catch the name? No? Why? Was your mind filled with other things, like the impression you were making or what you were going to say? Most people love to hear their own names and feel highly complimented when others remember them. Catching a name during an introduction is simply a matter of practice. Rather than be nervous about what to think or say, concentrate on the moment, for the only thing of importance in it is hearing the person's name. Quiet your mind and listen for it. If you don't catch it, ask for it to be repeated (people usually don't mind doing that at all), and then use it yourself when you reply: "How do you do, Maggie. My name is Janet." By vocalizing the name, your mind registers it much more firmly than it will if you try to register it mentally.

EYE CONTACT

With the name clearly in mind, look the person in the eyes. What color are they? What do you see in them? Does he or she look away? Eye contact is the most telling form of communication. You can learn much about what strangers are like merely by watching their eyes, as well as being aware of your own.

Because eye contact is learned from our parents, messages can get complicated and even distorted. On the one hand, children are rarely satisfied that they have the parent's attention until they get eye contact. Every parent knows that if two children are crying, the one who stops first is the one who gets the eye contact. On the other hand, parents may never give their children their full attention unless they are angry. How many times have you heard the phrase, spoken in outrage, "Look at me when I talk to you!" That's a negative form of reinforcement, and many children who heard it from their parents growing up give eye contact only when they fight. A lot of people actually have to look away to express their feelings and their deeper thoughts.

You can tell a lot about what feelings and thoughts people are having by watching what their eyes are doing. Looking up and to the right means they are trying to remember or put together an image or a picture. Looking up and to the left means they're trying to construct a picture or an image. Looking down and to the right is about attaching feeling to something. Looking down and to the left is about internal dialogue. Usually when people are feeling bad about themselves that's how I can tell. I know they're listening to the dialogues they're having with themselves.

If the eyes are at eye level and they look to the right, they're getting in touch with a song they've heard before, such as trying to remember the words of a song. If they're looking eye level and then to the left, they're trying to construct a sound, as my son does when he's trying to write music. There's so much being communicated by eye contact. Much of it we know inside, but we don't *know* what we know.

If you want to establish real intimacy with people, look into their eyes when you talk to them, and look into their eyes when you listen to them. Don't stare or you'll spook them, but if you are truly in search of being real with people, they will respond. In fact, they will open up and tell you things that are meaningful to them. Conversations will suddenly be easy because you won't be having to search for superficialities. People are yearning to get beneath the surface of things. Give them half a chance and they'll be grateful for it.

VOICE IMAGE

Anorexics and some bulimics have a special problem with voice image. One of the most common characteristics of the addiction is a tiny, childlike voice. When they say they can't understand why everyone treats them like a child, I say, "Because you speak like a child." Their voices come out of the top of the throat rather than resonated from the mouth, throat, and chest. No one wants to strain to listen. The metaphor of anorexia is a desire to disappear, and this includes vocally. Making an effort to be heard will diminish the power of that metaphor, and the encouraging feedback received from others will encourage the anorexic to reappear.

TOUCHING

In this dangerous age we live in, physical contact has become far less acceptable than in previous decades. Yet, people still yearn for closeness, and there are many ways to touch that demonstrate caring in a nonthreatening way. The safest place to touch someone is on the forearm. Its close proximity to the fingers, which deal with expression of thought rather than sexuality, makes it a safe place to make physical contact. To most people a touch on the forearm means emphasis, either in understanding or in reply to what has just been said.

Many females, however, feel violated if a man touches them on the upper arm, particularly if it is bare. I think the reason is a lot of women hide their breasts by crossing their arms, and touching the upper arm is tantamount to touching their breasts. If you don't want to offend a woman you've just met, touch her on the forearm. The shoulder is also an inoffensive place to touch. I have found in therapy sessions that if I touch someone on the stomach, all of a sudden they'll start expressing feelings. It's interesting to me that the stomach is the closest to food.

HUGS

A lot of people don't know how to give a proper hug. To me the best hug is eye contact first, to register intimacy, then a simple and spontaneous embrace with body contact coupled with loving thoughts. Pats on the back are for burping babies. The A-frame hug, with lots of space between the bodies, is a halfhearted affair. Then there's the "right boob, left boob" hug. Men have a tendency to hug that way, especially tall men. It's probably a variation of the embrace that features a peck on both cheeks. To me it's a busy hug, and too complicated. Why not just stand still and enjoy it?

In my years of therapy I've found it's the rare person who doesn't like to be hugged, and that person is inevitably the one who needs it the most. At the center, I don't give hugs just for shakes. I think some people have to be direct and ask for hugs, because that's one of the things people need to learn—to start going after what they want—but if I want to hug spontaneously, I feel free to do so.

It may seem simplistic to you at this point that developing social skills will make the difference between relapse and recovery, but I am convinced the reason Janet Greeson's "A Place For Us" is so successful is we're a treatment center that sends people out into the world knowing how to be social beings. People can go into treatment and successfully lose or gain weight, but what difference does that make if they go back out into society still feeling cold and numb and isolated, unable to communicate with others in a meaningful way? Real recovery is about changing lifestyle. Practicing basic social skills will do more for your future happiness than any calorie counter, and they're a lot more fun.

Workbook for Day Three

ASSIGNMENT ONE: DRAW YOUR FAMILY TREE

Label each member of your family and give them a grade that evaluates their social skills. High grades mean they had many close friends and long-term relationships, and that those social skills were passed on to you. Low grades mean few friends and long-term relationships. Write a few paragraphs about what you have learned about your family from doing this exercise and how they influenced your ability to communicate with intimacy.

ASSIGNMENT TWO: MEDITATION EXERCISE

Meditation is an important part of the Janet Greeson's "A Place For Us." When people begin to abstain from their compulsive eating patterns, the pain that coping mechanism had been masking begins to rise. Meditation is a spiritual alternative for dealing with the discomfort of those feelings.

Pain is a necessary part of change, but suffering is optional. As people experience the pain that comes with abstinence, they want to react to it, as that is what they have always done in the past. Reaction to pain is called suffering. Meditation is an alternative coping mechanism that allows the uncomfortable feelings to flow out of you without resisting them, thereby eliminating the need to suffer. Disengaging yourself from the pain of those percolating feelings takes away their power and the resulting suffering that has driven you to compulsive eating.

Early in your abstinence, when you feel overwhelmed with a sense of discomfort—a diffuse, all-encompassing dread, a feeling that life can't go on—it means the emotions you have been burying deep in your unconscious are beginning to rise. Later they will become more specific, but for now they are not truly observable and can be regarded as negative energy that needs to be discharged. Meditation is the conductor of that energy, allowing it to leave you while safely grounding you in a state of awareness in which you remain apart from the feelings, claiming them but not engaging them. It is a purifying process that will soon seem effortless.

The time to meditate is every time the compulsion to return to your destructive eating patterns returns. That compulsion may leave you in as little as a few minutes if you are able to quiet your mind. It is also a good idea to meditate at a certain time each day, such as early in the morning, during breaks in your working day, or in the evening. You don't need to spend more than a few minutes meditating. Five minutes will seem long in the beginning. Later you will find fifteen minutes and eventually a half hour passing without being aware of the time.

"Prayer is when we speak; meditation is when we listen." It's that simple. Meditation doesn't have to be mystical or ritualistic. It merely ceases the endless debates that go on in your head and allows you to be at one with yourself. It helps you escape the boundaries of noise and confusion and puts you on a new plane. In deep meditation you exist simultaneously at different levels of consciousness. Scientists have no way of explaining how a person can be in two different places at the same time, but people who practice meditation don't need an explanation. They feel it. What they are feeling is an increase in serotonin, the "feel good" hormone in the brain.

When people first start to meditate, they are often frustrated because they really become aware of the board meetings going on in their heads. They're supposed to be the chairman of that board, but they seem to have no control over the conversations and the confusion. You can stop all the chatter by focusing on your breathing:

Fill your lungs deeply, using your diaphragm muscles, taking in air to a slow count of eight or ten, and then releasing it all at once—let it go without holding it back. As you let it out, direct the air to where the chatter is and blow it away. When thoughts come into your mind, let them pass without resistance. Don't get frustrated when these thoughts resurface. It's your mind's job to think, and thoughts never stop; they just don't have to be owned. Listen not to them but to the silence in the background, for a message that has yet to come. Soon your thoughts will become the background, just another environmental irritant to ignore, and you will sink to another level of consciousness where you become quiet and at peace.

You will learn to love this state of mind, and to want to repeat the experience. In later exercises you will be given specific tasks to perform while meditating, visualizations that will lead you deeper and deeper into this altered state of consciousness. For today, just enjoy the silence. Set five minutes as your goal, and repeat those five minutes several times throughout the day.

A Day in the Life

TONY

Wednesday, 9:30 A.M. Finally got confirmation from Estelle on that Kansas City variance. If I hadn't kept the pressure up from here, the whole deal would have fallen through. How the hell am I going to hold everything together from here? It was insane to get myself talked into coming here. Every problem I have could be solved right now by leaving on the next available flight. Last night when I talked to Dad and told him I hadn't unpacked yet, he said, "Remember when you did three weeks for contempt of court?" Of course I did, my finest hour in some respects, standing up to that lousy judge on a case that was reversed on appeal. "Well," said Dad, "think of your present situation the same way." So I am. I'm doing time, counting the days until I get out of here. At least I'll lose weight in the process.

Noon. Walked twice around the fitness course and it felt good. Want to write down something Smitty said this morning in class about our heads being like a garbage bag stuffed too full. Add more trash and it keeps building up the pressure on the bag until it rips. That's a nervous breakdown, and the garbage comes out the wrong end. In group therapy the trash is taken out a piece at a time, examined, and discarded. I've had two sessions of group therapy with him so far and it's scary as hell. This one woman really let loose her anger yesterday. I felt bad for her, but I also wanted to bolt out of the room. Just don't want to examine the trash I've got in my head, I guess. Maybe after a few days when I get to know everybody a little better. The problem is, these people here have really serious problems, nothing like mine.

4:30 P.M. Talked to my son. Promised him a telescope if he passes the history test. The kid hates history. Hates school. Hates me, I think. The wife sounds frantic. Says I've got to call my sister because she's weeping and wailing and talking about jumping out the window.

10:30 P.M. Telephoned my sister and tried to calm her down. That bastard ex-husband of hers had been back for his summer clothes. He and his lady love are taking a cruise! I'd like to kill him with my bare hands. Told my sister she's got to pull herself together for the sake of her kids. What if they hear her talking about committing suicide? That sort of brought her to her senses. I'm exhausted. I'm supposed to be doing all this reading, and except for keeping up in this diary, I'm not doing any of the stuff I'm supposed to be doing. This meeting we went to tonight though was good. I heard a lot of things that I related to, like not being conscious of what I was putting in my mouth and feeling like I had to solve the problems of the world. Why is that? It was really good to get out of this place, riding the bus like a bunch of high schoolers on the way to a tournament. Passing every conceivable kind of fast-food restaurant on earth on the way, plus some I've never heard of, and enjoying the fact that I'm safe from temptation. One more phone call to the West Coast and I'm calling it a day.

Day Four

STEP STUDY: STEP ONE

(To get the most out of Step Study, buy or borrow a copy of *Alcoholics Anonymous* (the *Big Book*), published by Alcoholics Anonymous World Services, Inc. It's inexpensive and can be purchased at 12-step meeting places. The word "food" can be substituted for the word "alcohol" every time it appears in the text.) The Twelve Steps are reprinted and adapted throughout with permission of Alcoholics Anonymous World Services, Inc. The AA original Twelve Steps are reprinted in their entirety at the end of the book. Read "The Doctor's Opinion" and Chapter One, "Bill's Story," in the *Big Book*.

THE FIRST STEP: "We admitted we were powerless over food—that our lives had become unmanageable."

Admitting powerlessness is a devastating thing. We are brought up to be competitive and believe that saying we can't win is a sign of weakness. Admitting powerlessness is an act of letting go, which is the opposite of the struggle we've been in for so long, a 180-degree turnaround in thought and action. The struggle has been one of mortal combat for our very souls, and it has been unceasing, a twenty-four-hour-a-day battle without respite, even in sleep. We can wake up in the middle of the night and not know why we're awake. We're not hungry, but our thoughts are on the contents of the refrigerator.

We are engaged in struggle against an adversary that is "cunning, baffling, and powerful," that we can't see, can't really get in touch with, and the moment we let down our guard, it has a way of grabbing a new toehold, pushing harder against us. Every time we think we know something about it, we find out we don't know anything at all, but we keep on trying to win.

As long as we keep up the struggle against the addiction we will lose, for we are only playing into its power. The struggle connects us with the addiction and it will always win, and the prize is our very lives. Our bodies are the battleground and we are stuck there, connected to our addiction and in its viselike grip, as long as we continue to struggle. As soon as we surrender to our powerlessness we are free to remove ourselves from the battleground and live like normal people—if not a normal, everyday life, at least one in which we are not constantly distracted by the need to struggle.

Let's look at the problem in retrospect. What has fighting won you so far? Take a look at what your success has been in beating this addiction your way. You may have had times when you seemed to be making progress, and then in a moment, as soon as you let down your guard—perhaps went to a wedding and had a tiny sliver of cake, or were feeling blue and bought yourself a treat—faster than you could say "Hostess Twinkie" the addiction had you back down on your knees.

It's not your fault for being in the condition you are today. No amount of willpower can be used against an addiction that can't be outwitted or outmaneuvered.

If you still deny your problem has anything to do with being addicted but merely your inadequate self-will, remember that no one has more willpower over food than anorexics, and they lose the battle, too. Everyone loses as long as they continue to struggle, for an addiction that goes untreated gets progressively worse, never better.

Acceptance of powerlessness doesn't happen overnight. It moves through stages, from denial to anger to bargaining to depression and finally surrender. It is a process you may already be in, experiencing all these feelings. That is a good sign; it means you are engaged in the process and beginning to give up the struggle.

After denial comes anger; who wants to have a chronic and incurable addiction? The trouble is, we addicts don't know how to constructively express anger and make it work for us. We are accustomed to venting anger in dysfunctional acting out, usually by more compulsive eating. You may also experience scattershot anger—at everyone and everything, including this book. That's okay. Go for it. Anger is energy and needs to be discharged. Just don't express it in a way that harms yourself or others. Feelings of "It isn't fair!" and "What did I do to deserve this?" are legitimate but not helpful. You will move through them, so be patient with your state of mind and know it is part of the healing process.

Old angers may also emerge, over all the times you have been humiliated because of a condition you are beginning to realize is not your fault, over all the dances you didn't go to, the cliques that shunned you, the love affairs you didn't have. Honor these feelings. Don't try to numb or minimize them, no matter how much they hurt. They belong to you and need to be acknowledged.

After anger comes a renewal of denial: instead of struggling, you vow to negotiate with the addiction. You will follow a diet to the gram and will not snack in between meals. You will fast three days a week, eat normally three days, and binge on Sunday. You will enroll in a gym, go on a liquid-protein diet, run three miles a day—all to no avail. The bargaining period is one last desperate attempt to live a "normal" life, and failure to conjure up the needed willpower will land you in the next phase of the surrender process: depression. Look at it as a gift. You are almost there.

You have lots of reasons to feel depressed. You are losing your best friend and constant companion: food. You are facing the prospect of having to change, and no one relishes that. Your future is uncertain. You are afraid. Acknowledge all these feelings, too. Denying them will only make you more depressed. Be good to yourself in this phase and begin to take the actions that will lead you to recovery—in spite of your state of mind.

Acceptance is the final phase of the process, and at first it will seem unnatural: "Who cares to admit complete defeat? Practically no one, of course. Every natural instinct cries out against the idea of personal powerlessness." But believe me, the only way we can win is to surrender. When people balk at that idea, they forget they have already lost their will—to their addiction—for the progression of the addiction is a gradually diminished capability to exercise free will over use. Surrender is getting it back.

On page 448 of the *Big Book* a physician describes the phenomenon as follows: "After I had been around A.A. for seven months . . . I was finally able to say, 'Okay, God. It *is* true that I . . . really, really am a [food addict] of sorts. And it's all right with me. Now, what am I going to do about it?' When I stopped living in the problem and began living in the answer, the problem went away. From that moment on, I have not had a single compulsion to [overeat]."

When you finally stop fighting and loosen the desperate grip you hold on the addiction, the addiction inexplicably and miraculously loosens its desperate grip on you, and you can begin the journey of recovery. Surrender places the addict in you under house arrest, one day at a time. Remember, the person who got up the earliest this morning is the one with the longest sobriety. Every addict needs to surrender every day. It's the nature of the recovery process.

There are people who stop working the program at the point their compulsion is lifted. You may know alcoholics who quit drinking using the "white knuckle" approach, without working an Anonymous program. Although they were abstinent, their behavior remained the same. They didn't drink anymore, but they were still self-centered and egotistical and miserable most of the time, having denied themselves the one comfort they had found in life. Food addicts can also have abstinence without recovery. But recovery is about becoming "happy, joyous, and free." If you want that, too, you need to work a 12-step program.

The admission of powerlessness must be complete. The text describes how in the early years of AA "none but the most desperate cases" could commit themselves to such a program. Those whose lives had not yet reached the point of utter unmanageability continued to believe that somehow, somewhere, someday, they were going to beat the addiction. They were destined to go through the addiction process to its final stages of living hell, at which time they would reach out for the program like "the drowning seize life preservers." That has changed today. Many people come into 12-step programs now before they've reached that bitter "low bottom" point.

The text warns those who haven't hit their bottom, get introduced to the twelve steps, and then decide to try more controlled eating: "When one [food addict] has planted in the mind of another the true nature of his malady, that person can never be the same again." You might go out and try using your best effort to control your eating just out of sheer rebellion and anger, but it will never be the same as it was. Your guilt will be twice as guilty, and your pain will be twice as painful. Before you read this book you probably didn't know there was an answer, or that the condition you're in is not your fault.

But once you understand the nature of the addiction and know how you can get better, if you go out and start participating in the addiction again, it's by conscious choice. When you know what you can do and won't do it, then you do become responsible for the condition you're in. You may still have to do it your way, and that's all right. Some food addicts have to get to the point of sheer hopelessness before they surrender. If you are one, just remember when you reach that point, you can resume your journey into recovery.

If you would like to save yourself the pain of testing your will against the disease of food addiction one more time, that, too, is your choice. If you have suffered enough, you can let go now of that deathlike grip on the end of your rope and after a few initial moments of panic, experience a joyful free-fall into sanity.

Workbook for Day Four

ASSIGNMENT ONE: YOUR CASE HISTORY

The story of Bill W., pages 1 through 16 in the *Big Book*, is a case history of addiction, covering a twelve-to-fifteen-year period from the beginning to the final stages of the disease, and shows the progression of alcohol in his life.

Write a case history of your food addiction, showing how it has affected your life, drawing parallels to Bill W.'s story. Begin with the time in your life when food first became a problem and end it with where you are now and your hopes and plans for today.

A Day in the Life
ELAINE

Thursday. 8 A.M. My head is throbbing something fierce. I can't believe how painful this withdrawal is. I feel like I've been filling my body with poison, and now that it's leaving my system it's letting me know how much harm it's been doing to me. I just can't wait until I'm detoxified. Sugar, you are so bad! Or maybe it's the caffeine. Who knows at this point? I'm almost grateful that I got the bad news about my son when I'm already in such pain a little more couldn't make much of a difference. Danny called my husband last night to say he had been arrested for driving while intoxicated, second offense, so he's had his license taken away. Now he has to get to work by taking a bus and is looking for a job closer to his apartment. Why do I react to these problems my grown children have as though they were my fault? What could I have done that I didn't do already? My husband tried to console me. Says some people have to learn by their mistakes and that Danny's essentially a good kid, just needs to stop drinking and drugging. That gets me all riled up again. What drugs? I want to know, but my husband tries to get off the hook. He's broken a confidence he says. I bet it's cocaine. That would explain why Danny's always short of money. I just feel so awful. And this afternoon we're having psychodrama, which one of the patients laughingly calls "emotional sandblasting." Terrific. Just what I need.

11 A.M. I walked with Kathryn, who's in my group therapy. On Monday she did what's called anger work here, and I told her I'm amazed to see the difference in her. She's childlike now—that's the only way I can describe it—peaceful instead of anguished. Her face was all pinched and pained before. Now it's open. She looks ten years younger. She tells me she felt sick all day yesterday,

like getting all that anger out of her was also like a detox. She hugged me. She's so frail. I could feel all her bones and felt so huge. Tears came to my eyes. "You'll be all right," she told me. "Just trust this place. I was like you when I came in." I asked her what she meant by that and she just smiled.

3 P.M. I'm weak from psychodrama. It was really something. When we count off and break up into smaller groups. I get a different counselor, Vickie. She asks us to act out the happiest day of our lives. I enact leaving home for college, others their wedding day, birth of a child, this very pretty woman Jean when she won a beauty contest. Then they pass around big sheets of paper and felt-tip markers and ask us to draw the saddest day of our lives. I thought for a while, getting sad just thinking about all the opportunities—the affair, my son's DWI, my father's funeral—but then I remembered something I hadn't thought about in years, when my dog got hit by a truck. Just drawing it I started to sob, remembering those silly brown and black spots and that trusting look in his eyes, the way he sighed so peacefully in my arms when I felt the life go out of him. When I told the story to my group, I cried harder than I've ever cried in my life over the loss of that silly dog. "What's going on for you?" Vickie said. I felt so foolish. "That dog loved me so," I blurted out. "He was always so glad to see me."

"What else was going on in your life at that time?" Vickie asked me.

"My dad died!" I was really mortified to put those two events together. Here I'd put the loss of my dog before the loss of my father as my saddest memory, but everyone else was too absorbed in their own pain to pay much attention.

Then Kathryn showed us a picture of herself as a little girl looking out her bedroom window waiting for her daddy to drive by in his car and wave at her, which he did every night about nine o'clock she said, and I knew the whole story was just her fond imagining. I started crying all over again, thinking of this child standing by the window in her little pajamas waiting for a daddy who never came.

Afterward we put all our drawings in the middle of

the floor, they were covered up with a sheet, and we stood in a circle sobbing over our loved ones, our griefs, our losses, all in a sad pile under the sheet while music played in the background. Then when I didn't think there was another drop of tears left in me, Blanche brought us back to reality by making up play a silly nursery game and we laughed like little kids. Then everybody went around hugging each other. It felt good, and safe, even with the men. By the time we went to Wellness lecture we were in a hilarious mood. It was such a powerful experience. Crying in front of other people isn't easy, but when everybody does it, it's okay, almost like natural. Where else in the world do people not hide their tears or go cry alone? We're not supposed to do that here. I remember all the crying I've done in the shower because no one can hear me there—crying with no comfort in it.

3 P.M. Wellness lecture with Ken. He says, "I'm a neo-anthropological archaeologist digging among the living for buried treasure." We laugh when he tells us he's wacko, too, but he gets to go home. He says he likes to work with people in treatment centers because they're honest.

9 P.M. I'm feeling down again. I thought my withdrawal headache was gone and now it's back. There's such cliquishness here. I'm so lonely. I try to get close to people by being helpful, but when I sat on the bus tonight and there was an empty seat next to me and the others piled in and no one came to sit by me, I felt like no one here really likes me. There was all this hilarity going on all around but I didn't feel a part of it. I've always felt that way, especially in a crowd. Why is that? Why don't people seek me out? Why do I have to seek *them* out? And why did I have to get such a mean roommate? She's so angry. Even her hair is angry, bristling all around her face. She left wet towels all over the bathroom floor again. I begged Smitty to get put in with someone else and he told me, "If you can't work out problems you have with other people here, you never will on the outside," and then goes on about boundaries. I was really mad at him but didn't say anything. I want to go home!

Day Five

IDENTIFYING AND VALIDATING YOUR FEELINGS

Food addicts have learned to turn off their feelings, or bury them under layers of fat. Mostly what they feel is numb. My job is to get you to feel again, so you won't have to use food to medicate those emotions you haven't been able to handle any other way. Rather than deal with feelings that come from events that happened to you long ago, I want to focus on the feelings you have today, the results of events that are happening now. Maybe someone vented a lot of anger at you in an inappropriate way, or you were put down by a person you love. These are the feelings that are the most readily identifiable, and you need practice validating and expressing them in ways that make you feel competent about yourself. Competency has a lot to do with being able to tune in on what is happening to you in the moment, not trying to understand what happened to you long ago.

First, let's focus on identifying feelings. That may sound simplistic, but a lot of food addicts have denied their feelings so thoroughly they don't even know what they are anymore. They believe thinking is a feeling because they live in their heads. If you can substitute the words "I think" for "I feel," what you're describing is not a feeling. For example, "I feel this is an uplifting experience" is a judgment, not a feeling. However, if you can substitute "I am" for "I feel," you are in the realm of feelings. The words "I am lonely" are one and the same. Simple adjectives and adverbs are required, not clauses preceded by "I feel that." You see how avoiding feelings is built right into the sentence structure of people who find them too threatening to express.

Feelings are most readily identified when they are a spontaneous response to something that happened in the present. Think of an occasion recently when someone said or did something to which you responded by feeling awful. Did you ignore those painful feelings, hoping they would go away, or tell yourself you must have done something to deserve it? The first thing to acknowledge is the fact that you have a feeling at all, and describe it to yourself, know that what you're experiencing is true to you. If your truth is questioned, be willing to bear the pain of someone else's not understanding. It's *you* who needs to validate your reality.

In the acknowledgment stage, it doesn't help a bit to analyze what's going on inside, asking yourself, "I feel this way because . . ." If someone walks over and stomps on your toe, your toe doesn't care if it was done on purpose or by accident! The first step of recovery is knowing your toe hurts! Why it hurts is not important, or asking, is it all right for my toe to hurt? Or, should it hurt this much? Or, is it my fault that it hurts? Or, what could I have done so that this wouldn't have happened? *Know* it hurts so you can take care of it! The obviousness of that acknowledgment is not at all simplistic. How many times has someone caused you pain and then said, "That didn't hurt" or "This hurts me a lot worse than it does you"? There are a lot of bullies in this world who use the tactic of denial to confuse people when they're in the midst of dealing with their pain. Analyzing it continues the short circuit. What's important is that *you* know you're in pain, and that's all the validation you need.

So there you are: Someone has just had an anger binge and dumped on you. You feel mixed up, scared, confused, angry, and depressed. In your mind you acknowledge your feelings. You skip "should," "ought," and "fault" and say, "Wow. I really feel mixed up, scared, confused, angry, and depressed." Notice you have *described* the experience to yourself, not *evaluated* it. If someone else does, and says something like, "You're not handling this very well" or "Don't worry. You'll be fine," you may want to respond, but stick to describing the experience: "Excuse me, I'd like to respond to that, but at the moment I'm overwhelmed." When you're out of control in a feeling, it's not the time to figure things out.

Sometimes people are pressed into making decisions in a distressed state because they don't realize they have the option *not* to respond when their feelings are out of control. They have the right to buy time by saying things like, "I don't know" or "I'll get back to you" or "I don't want to say right now." All these replies allow you time to process your feelings before taking action. Every time feelings of anger, confusion, or anxiety rise in you because people are bulldozing you, that is your cue to take care of your feelings, not react to the prodding.

It's also not the time to get combative. If you respond to someone's temper trantrum by telling them they don't have a right to dump their anger on you, you get involved in a moral issue, which is bound to lead to an argument. You're not up to that right now, confused as you are in the midst of dealing with your pain. What would you do if they were to angrily reply, "I don't get my rights from you. And furthermore . . ." The only rights you can focus on are your own rights, and the only person who is responsible for your own rights is you.

I heard a colleague of mine tell a story about a man who used to take out all his anger and frustration on Jewish people. One day he passed a rabbi on the street and made an ugly comment. The rabbi said, "Wait a minute."

"Yeah? What?" said the man.

"Is that all?" said the rabbi.

"No!"

"What else have you got to say?"

More garbage spewed forth. The rabbi kept asking "What else?" until the man had used up all the ugly things he could say. Then the rabbi said, "If I came over to your house and dumped all my garbage in your driveway, what would you do?"

The man said, "I'd have it hauled out. I don't need any of your garbage."

"That's right," said the rabbi, "and I'm leaving your garbage right here," and walked away.

Leaving the ugly words behind and walking away is a declaration of your rights, and a good choice in your state—you can't think and feel at the same time. When you declare your own rights, you have established an internal criterion that can't be taken away by someone else.

As you walk away, you can seek out a safe place to process your feelings. If you're in a situation where it's difficult to walk away, such as from an angry boss in an office, there's always a readily available and acceptable "safe place"—the bathroom. On your way, you can begin to reestablish your equilibrium by getting connected to your hurt feelings in a positive way. Are they connected to the fact that you care so much that you hurt? Are they connected to the fact that you have a very high sense of personal integrity and your life doesn't work well when you can't match it? Those are valuable attributes you have chosen to have. When you can't make sense of the big picture, you need to come back to the small part of the world that is you and say, "Okay, what can I do right now that would be useful, based on my values and who I am?" You need a reference, or you may enter into that state of free-floating anxiety that happens when people can't find one.

That state is common these days. We live in a world of relative values and uncertain morality. Everyone is struggling with these issues and no one seems to have the answers, lacking any kind of standardized frame of reference. Religious sources are supposed to offer a moral reference, but often only add to the confusion. I heard about a woman who got terribly depressed because she had been listening to a tape that told her, "You'll know a person is a Christian by the fruits she's bearing," and she said, "But I'm not bearing any fruit. I must not be a Christian." I don't know much about that, but I know that orange trees don't bear fruit all year. What season was she in?

Free-floating anxiety is anxiety that doesn't have a reference, and it's likely to be the state you're in as you walk away from an unpleasant experience. You need some immediate orientation, starting with who you are right now, where you are, and what's true for you, and to forget about establishing references outside yourself. In your state, if you spend a lot of time trying to know more about what you're scared of before you get a reference, your free-floating anxiety can develop into stormy anxiety, a form of unintentional self-hypnosis, such as when you were a kid and spent the night together with other kids telling ghost stories. After a couple of hours you couldn't go to sleep!

Self-hypnosis is the loss of sensory awareness of the here and now. Anytime you're out of control, you're under self-hypnosis. You are in a stuck state and need to get unstuck. Unless you get out of it, your anxiety will trigger other negative responses, almost phobic in nature, vestigial memories of every other time in your life you've felt powerless and victimized, then judging yourself for having the feelings in the first place. Words such as "stupid" and "dumb" and "how could you?" and images of other failures will soon have you immobilized.

If you lose yourself once more in the painful event, look at it as if it were a movie on your VCR and fast-forward it to the end. Then run it backward. If it were a war movie, it would start with the mushroom cloud and end with the uranium being put back in the mines. You can defuse the event in the same way. The terror of a traumatic event is the loss of self. If you can maintain orientation, you can deal with the problem and not the loss of power.

Remember, you are no longer doomed to remain in the stuck state that comes with denial of feelings. You have honored them and are now free to move out of that state into a competent one. Your first task is to ground yourself in the present moment. Become aware of stimuli that are not involved in your tension. A telephone rings, a horn honks outside your window, a baby cries. Orient yourself to the space you're in, feel what you're touching, observe what you're seeing. Be in the now so you aren't in every other situation that's made you feel this way, particularly the ones from your childhood when you were truly helpless. You're not that now. You're a competent adult and you've got new tools to deal with these situations that used to make you so afraid.

Now that you are firmly grounded in the present, you need to reframe, not reblame. You need to ask yourself not the old question of "Whose fault is it?" but "What do I need?" Objectivity? Strength? Detachment? A relaxed state of mind? Flexibility and balance? Humor? When you have answered that question for yourself, ask another: "Where did I have that?" Put yourself into a situation where you had it and feel the power and the creativity of that moment. If you can't find a situation in which you were able to give yourself what you needed, visualize giving it to yourself now. Then run the sequence of the unpleasant event that just happened, freeze-frame, step into the scene, put your arms around yourself, and give yourself what you need. That's called reframing.

By using our feelings as a guide rather than a hindrance, we can learn to deal with the here and now. The origins of those feelings may never be discovered, and even if they are, they might not make any difference in how you cope with your present life. Merely acknowledging them and loving yourself for having them is a healthy beginning. The rest is practice.

Workbook for Day Five

ASSIGNMENT ONE: DESCRIBING FEELINGS

Search your memory and record an event, major or recent, when you have experienced the following emotions:

Close________________ Distant________________

Powerful________________ Submissive________________

Independent________________ Insecure________________

Talkative________________ Quiet________________

Cooperative________________ Angry________________

Firm________________ Evasive________________

Self-assured________________ Embarrassed________________

Seductive________________ Contemptuous________________

Open________________ Aggressive________________

Happy________________ Anxious________________

Calm________________ Sad________________

Confident________________ Fearful________________

Warm________________ Guilty________________

Excited________________

Breathless________________

Soft________________

Relaxed________________

Appealing________________

Determined________________

Surprised________________

Ecstatic________________

Grateful________________

Strong________________

Affectionate________________

Lighthearted________________

Compassionate________________

Proud________________

Comforted________________

Hopeful________________

Tolerant________________

Carefree________________

Respectful________________

Tender________________

Sexy________________

Silly________________

Peaceful________________

Enraged________________

Panicky________________

Timid________________

Dishonest________________

Two-faced________________

Choked up________________

Numb________________

Locked in________________

Belligerent________________

Vacant________________

Depressed________________

Immobilized________________

Tense________________

Horrified________________

Threatened________________

Beaten________________

Lonely________________

Weepy________________

Resentful________________

Envious________________

Confused________________

Powerless________________

Inadequate________________

Thrilled________	Torn________
Contented________	Debased________
Thankful________	Bored________
Pleased________	Impatient________
Courageous________	Jealous________
Frisky________	Spineless________

You will notice that the positive feelings appear in the left-hand column and the negative feelings in the column on the right. Go over what you have written and look for patterns. Do certain people, places, and things keep appearing in your descriptions? If so, what?________
Based on what you find, evaluate which situations, actions, and persons give you pleasure and which cause you pain.________

____

Was it difficult for you to get in touch with your feelings?

____

If so, which ones?________
What have you learned about yourself as a feeling person from taking this inventory?________

ASSIGNMENT TWO: MEDITATION EXERCISE

Lie comfortably and begin breathing deeply, taking in the breath slowly and letting it all out at once. Beginning at your toes and working up, be aware of how your body feels. Wherever you feel some discomfort, cup your hands over the area, look at your cupped hands, and ask, "What is this pain about?" If you do this exercise with full concentration, your mind will interpret the answer your body gives it.

A Day in the Life
JEAN

7 A.M. I actually woke up hungry. That hasn't happened to me in years. Yesterday I really had the urge to throw up after putting away that afternoon snack of cheese and crackers, but my roommate would have heard me. I hear other treatment centers monitor their bulimics a lot closer, locking the bathrooms for two hours after they eat and things like that. We get told over and over we have to assume responsibility for ourselves. Nobody's going to stand over us and tell us to eat. Still, there's no privacy here. Jill is a good roommate, very warm and motherly, and I don't want to upset her. If there was only a quiet way to throw up.

I take an early-morning walk with Tim. The sky is purple, opalescent, and the trees look French. When I feel stronger, we're going to jog every morning before breakfast. I think my detox headache is starting to lift.

I don't like group therapy. For one thing, there's this real angry person named Gloria in my group. I don't like her and she makes it clear she doesn't like me. Other people in the group complain about her a lot, but not to her face. Yesterday I told Blanche that I want to deal with my problems in individual sessions with her, and she says I need to bring my problems to group and deal with them there. I don't like her either. She dresses too prissily. I'm having trouble trusting her. My feelings about this place are deteriorating.

Community meeting. Now I'm really mad. We got chewed out for coming late to meetings. They also want us to wear shoes and it's more comfortable to go barefoot. There's wall-to-wall carpeting and it's hot. I'm thinking, though, I guess lateness is passive-aggressive behavior. Guess what, my clock is now twenty minutes slow and I can't fix it.

1 P.M. Group therapy with Blanche. This woman who's leaving today, a bulimic and a cocaine addict, reads a letter to her dead boyfriend. When she was sixteen, he committed suicide and blamed her in the note he left. His mother slapped her face at the funeral, and someone

spray-painted her name on buildings around town calling her a murderess. She cried and cried. All this emotion really gets me down. Blanche asked me what was going on with me and I told her, "How can I take up the group's time talking about my problems? They're just so petty!" Blanche is very motherly but tough. She says there's a lot to get to when the tears come for others, and all of a sudden I'm just crying so hard and don't know why, which makes my head throb even worse. "Leave me alone!" I tell her.

3 P.M. I HATE IT HERE. I WANT TO LEAVE. I WANT TO GO HOME NOW. I'M BORED. I WANT PRIVACY. I HATE EVERYONE. EVERYTHING STINKS.

5 P.M. I'm better. I read this entry over and remember something I heard. When I say I'm bored, I'm really saying I'm afraid. Afraid of what? I ate dinner with Tim and he made me laugh.

10 P.M. My headache does not possess me. It is hovering, like a crab that has relaxed its claws. The OA meeting tonight was really supportive. A woman came in and cried so hard it was painful to watch. She said she had stopped drinking, taking cocaine, then cigarettes, and now she's bingeing on sugar. Said she ate three Hershey bars on the way to the meeting. She's gotten all these tickets for speeding, cracked up her car, just sobs and sobs. People in the room tell her she's come to the right place, that she's just like them, and that all that sugar is making her act crazy, but she runs out of the room bawling. Someone runs after her. When the meeting breaks up, just about everyone from the center surrounds her, hugging her, telling her to come to Janet Greeson's "A Place For Us." I feel so good. Two sayings I heard tonight that I like: "You can't feed an empty heart with a knife and fork" and "If you don't like what you hear, you can leave, but give us thirty days and if you don't like us, we'll gladly refund you your misery."

There was a lot of joking around the nurses' station tonight as we're eating our fruit. Linda, this very withdrawn anorexic, is eating her sandwich. Jill, my roommate, who's pretty hefty, says to her, "How much will you sell that sandwich for? A hundred dollars?" Then Tony, this hot-shot executive from New York, says, "Will you take Visa or MasterCard?" "Jewelry?" says Jill. Even Linda laughed.

10 P.M. I was writing this letter to my father I'm supposed to read aloud in group and crying and Elaine came in to see Jill. She saw I was crying and came into my space and started smothering me, making kiss noises, and I pushed her away. Some older women try to mother in such an offensive way. Elaine is such a phony, so cheerful all the time. Sometimes I wonder if she's just here to lose weight. Then Jill gave me Mexican turtle oil for my sunburn. That was nice. I feel comforted. Jill is gentle and respectful of my space. She's honest in her own pain. I don't care if I hurt Elaine's feelings. She's got to learn to be herself.

Day Six
EXPRESSING FEELINGS

Feelings are neither good nor bad. They just are. They're what we have the most of and know the least about. We can't control having them, but we can change them by modifying the way we respond to them. We channel them into action, not reaction.

Now that we have learned to identify and validate all those feelings we have been denying and medicating with food, what do we do with them? How can they be expressed to our advantage? Most likely, the old pattern has been a long simmer followed by a sudden outburst, which inevitably backfires and never gets us what we want. After feeling victimized for so long, when we finally express ourselves, we become the victimizer! Then, full of remorse and guilt, we go back into our shell and decide we are hopeless communicators.

There is hope. It lies in learning an entirely new mode of expression. We need to develop a new syntactical structure that will contain our feelings and still allow for thought. It is simple and involves six small words: "When you," "I feel," and "I need."

WHEN YOU . . .

Here is a hypothetical situation: Your mother interrupts you for the twenty-fourth time in a telephone conversation. Your stomach is churning over the years and years of enduring her interruptions, for all the times you have remained silent, for all the other indignities you have suffered because she doesn't listen to you, doesn't seemingly care what you have to say, doesn't want to hear about your hopes, dreams, fears, and ideas. After you hang up the telephone, you decide you will punish her by not calling her for a while. Weeks later, she calls you and berates you for neglect. You explode.

That's the old pattern.

Here is the new way you can express your feelings. You can practice it the next time someone who is significant to your life and purports to care about you says or does something that elicits hurt feelings. Note I didn't say "makes you feel bad" or "causes you pain." "Elicit" means to call up, to evoke, to draw forth, to bring up something potential or latent. Merely the voice tones of a significant person in your life can hit a childhood memory trace and put you back in the child state. The action of the other person has resulted in those feelings *that are already there* to emerge and be reexperienced.

As soon as you say "you" the other person will get defensive. When you respond by saying "You make me feel bad," the other person has every reason to say "What did I do that was so bad? You're always overreacting." Short of physical violence, another person can't "make" you feel bad. If the person interrupting you was someone you didn't care about or had no emotional hold over you, you might be annoyed or simply tell yourself not to seek out that person's company anymore. But it's your mother, and you're in turmoil, a seething mass of feelings. You care!

Begin your response by taking a deep breath and then letting it out. When people are in a feeling state they often forget to breathe. They take a sharp intake of breath and then hold it, under some kind of delusion that they are controlling themselves. This is no time to deny oxygen to your brain. Breathing space also gives time to collect your thoughts.

The first phase begins with the words "When you" and ends with an action: "When you interrupt me," "When you raise your voice," "When you give me unsolicited advice," "When you are late," "When you forget," "When you criticize me," "When you leave a mess in the kitchen"—whatever the present action is. Keep it to the incident that brought up the feelings, not all the other times it happened. "You always" and "You never" shut down communication and leave room for debate. Avoid extreme statements and stick to the present.

I FEEL . . .

The second phase is to learn to confront by saying "I feel." You can't be condemned for having feelings. They're yours and you have a right to them.

What *do* you feel? Angry? Insignificant? Humiliated? Afraid? Annoyed? Check the list of feeling words in yesterday's workbook if you're having difficulty identifying what you feel. If you can't bring yourself to make a barefaced emotional statement, try saying "I feel like": "When you interrupt me, I feel like what I have to say doesn't matter."

Maybe the other person will say, "I don't think your feelings are well-founded. You shouldn't feel that way." The response to that is, "But I do."

Notice the statement "I feel" does not talk about "you." Avoid that word and you will be amazed how much people will be able to hear you out. As soon as you start making "you" accusations, the other party is ready for a fight. Talking about yourself and your feelings disarms them. Instead of saying "When you don't listen to me, you make me so mad," say "When you turn on the TV while I'm talking to you, I feel ignored."

"But" negates whatever is stated prior to it, such as "I know you don't intend to be rude, but" or "You may not know this bothers me, but." That word crops up in communication all the time, and it's usually meant to soften the blow. Instead it gets in the way of communication.

You may find that your respectful statement of feelings produces no response at all, or wordless surprise or confusion at what to say. In that silence you can inject the third part of the response.

I NEED . . .

Rather than say "If only you would . . ." speak of your desires. It's disrespectful to say you want someone to change. Instead, express what you need from that person.

What *do* you need? Maybe you have never thought much about that before: "I need respect for my decisions." "I need someone to listen to me." "I need help." "I need understanding."

Making a simple statement about what you need moves the communication forward. Instead of veering toward accusation and blame, plus a round of nit-picking debate about the incident that provoked the confrontation, stating what you need offers a solution. You have given the person who has offended you a graceful way out of the confrontation, if he or she wants to take it. If not, what does that say about the person? It may be painful to realize that someone who means something to you isn't interested in meeting your needs, but it's better to know than to guess, and you have really cleared the air by your declaration.

You may not get what you want when you express your feelings, but you will feel powerful afterward. You have been honest, open, and direct. You will have respected yourself and other people enough to tell them what's going on with you. People will treat you with the same amount of respect as you command; you have been the role model of what you expect back, whether you get it or not.

Most of all, you will not have made a fool of yourself by sputtering and fuming, and then enduring the usual backlash. You will feel confident that you can communicate your feelings and needs again and again, and you will feel released from the terrible prison you have been in where you struggle with your feelings and never get them expressed to the outside world in a way that gets heard. Congratulations!

Workbook for Day Six

ASSIGNMENT ONE: WHEN YOU . . . I FEEL . . . I NEED

Recall the last time you either failed to express your feelings or botched the job with a significant person in your life—a spouse, lover, son or daughter, parent, friend, or neighbor. Focus on that situation now, and try to recall the exact words or actions that set you off. Write down what happened here: ______________________________

____

Now write the response you could have made or will make next time this situation occurs, beginning with the words "When you": ______________________________

Add the words "I feel" and describe your feelings:

____

Now add the statement, "I need": ______________

____

How do you feel about the statement you have just made? ______________________________________

ASSIGNMENT TWO: COMMITMENT

Make a commitment to yourself here that you will use this new way of expressing your feelings with this significant person in your life the next time it is appropriate to do so.

____

____

A Day in the Life

TONY

Saturday. On the weekends families come for therapy, and we had a group session this morning with all of us. It was really uncomfortable. I was glad no one from my family was down. I wanted to try to protect everyone's feelings, soothe things down. A woman patient and her sister really went at it. It was painful to watch but also wonderful to see them move from barely communicating to embracing each other. The sister was a real powerhouse—controlling, loud voice, dramatic gestures. The patient kept getting more and more withdrawn, then cried out in such agony when she had to come to grips with her enmeshment with her sister, how she was too close to her and let her rule her life. Underneath both of the exteriors sitting so stiffly next to each other were these two people crying out to be close. I kept thinking what would happen if anyone in my family came down. That would really turn into a free-for-all.

4 P.M. Elaine, Jill, my roommate Mike, and I go to a really dumb movie on our Saturday-afternoon pass. The women wanted to see it and I didn't care, just wanted to get out of the center and feel like a civilian again. I nearly passed out when I smelled the popcorn in the lobby, but none of us cheated. Can't see the point in that when we're committed to this program. Afterward we went to Friendly's and I had a diet soda, sitting there surrounded by all those color photographs of food, thinking of all the Friendly's I've binged in across the country. We traded pig-out stories and laughed our heads off. No one could top Jill's, about when she was in a hospital and had a blind roommate. She says she stole the cupcake off her dinner tray. I'm actually glad to be back here out of temptation's way. If I had been alone, I'm not at all sure I would have been able to pass that popcorn stand, let alone settle for a diet soda instead of a triple-fudge sundae. It's funny, though. The first few days here I lurked around the elevator before each meal, waiting for the trays to come up. Now I'm actually surprised to hear the bell. We hardly eat anything at all, but I'm not really hungry. Of course, I'm kind of under the weather detoxifying, and that helps. I don't drink coffee, so it must be sugar withdrawal.

6 P.M. Called home. My son flunked the history test. I started yelling at him and then stopped, remembering the assignment about "When you—I feel." Took a deep breath and said, "When you don't study, I feel bad." There was this long pause. "What's the matter, Dad? Are you okay?" he says. Then my wife gets on the line. "What did you say to him?" she says. I told her and she laughed. "What's so funny?" I ask. She says, "I don't know. I guess I've never heard you tell me or anyone how you feel." That really got me to thinking. "So, big deal," I

said, "I've got feelings, too. Is that such a surprise?" She got real serious then and said, "I know when you're angry, that's for sure. But come to think of it, I don't ever remember you expressing any feeling other than that." I tell her I love her.

10 P.M. OA meeting tonight. I actually said something. Can't remember what it was, but I got all choked up and couldn't finish. Two things I heard that really got to me: "One is too much, a thousand's not enough" and "You never have enough of what you don't want." But what do I really want? Peace of mind, for one thing. An end to all these troubles people keep dumping on me. Rode home on the bus with Mike, who's leaving next week. He's been in a program for a while and is full of the lingo, but he's a good guy. He tells me he thinks it's time I unpacked. I had to laugh at that. Didn't think he noticed!

Day Seven
SPIRITUALITY

The terrible emptiness addicts feel that they are compelled to fill with something outside themselves—a substance, activity, relationships—is the absence of their energy, spirit. Once they abstain from their obsession, that void can feel intolerable for a while. No matter where they go, they feel no one's there. Nothing they do or say is of any significance.

"A cup must be empty to be filled." Once it is drained of all illusions and false securities, it can be replenished, with your real spirit. The more expressive you become, the more spiritual you are. The essence of spirituality at Janet Greeson's "A Place For Us" is that we help people empty themselves so there is room for their spirit, their real energy, to fill the void. This is in no way a religious program. It's more about expression of energy. Birds sing, dogs bark. We are multifaceted expressions of energy. Religion is about dogma and ritual. Spirituality is about becoming positive, creative, loving, and enthusiastic human beings. The Greek derivation of the word "enthusiasm" is "God in me." That's the energy within you waiting to be tapped, waiting to be released.

I like to think of the word "God" as meaning "good orderly direction." The direction is not to follow a leader but the still, small voice that speaks to us when we listen, the light we see, the energy we express, the one we know without knowing is our higher self. Addiction is a detour away from that person, and recovery is a rediscovery of who we would have been, had our addiction not gotten in the way.

The Twelve Steps and Twelve Traditions of Alcoholics Anonymous says, "In every case, pain has been the price of admission into the new life." The intolerable pain of addiction compels people to seek a way other than their own, for it becomes obvious to them that their way is not working. Surrender of self-will is all that needs to be done to get in touch with a power higher than ourselves. That power will not come knocking on your door, but those who acknowledge their powerlessness are amazed at how readily it responds.

Surrender is not giving up but giving in—to make room for a powerful source of love and nurturance that will help you if you only ask. The miracle of this program is that we can change. We were not put on this earth to suffer but to be "happy, joyous, and free." A 12-step program is a blueprint for that. It has no leaders or holy gurus, no hierarchy, no promotional gimmicks. No one ever got rich or famous exploiting it. It does not even advertise that it exists, but people in pain find it and get better. You can, too.

The following is a prayer commonly used at 12-step meetings. It is identified with Christianity. Because it is so familiar, the meaning behind the words has lost its impact. I have supplied you with a meditation on what the words might mean to you.

THE LORD'S PRAYER

Our Father . . .

A genderless word, the source of unconditional love we may never have had from another human being, a parent to the needy child within us.

Which art in heaven . . .
Not a place in the sky or an afterlife, but now, within us, waiting to be occupied.

Hallowed be thy name . . .
As soon as the power of this source of universal love is made abstract by giving it a name, it can be abused by those who would claim it, proselytize, and brutalize others who call it by a different name.

Thy kingdom come . . .
To heal this suffering world we live in.

Thy will be done on earth as it is in heaven . . .
My will has enslaved me. Your will is to set me free.

Give us this day our daily bread . . .
Enough for today, no need for a surplus that can be hoarded, bought, and sold. One day at a time you give me all I need if I only ask, and tomorrow you will give again.

And forgive us our trespasses . . .
You don't speak of sins but of boundaries I have crossed.

As we forgive those who trespass against us . . .
Having been so readily forgiven by you for violating the boundaries of others, I return the favor. I hold no ill will in order to leave room for love.

And lead us not into temptation . . .
I am tested every day. You will lead me down another, safer path if I ask you every day.

But deliver us from evil . . .
You are there to protect me from the destructiveness of negativity, both within me and all around me. You will keep me safe if I ask you every day.

For thine is the kingdom . . .
Not mine, or anyone else's who seeks to own it, for it is not a place to be owned.

The power . . .

For You do not abuse it.

And the glory . . .

For which I freely give credit where it's due, to save myself from the enslavement of grandiosity.

Forever and ever . . .

The world will not come to an end. It will go through changes but it will not die.

Amen.

A Day in the Life

ELAINE

Sunday. Can't believe I've been here a week today. My headache is finally lifting. When I walked around the hospital this morning with Jill, I actually felt like I was here, felt the breeze on my cheeks and the sun beating down on my forehead. What a fog I've been in. Tomorrow we get weighed. I know I've dropped a few pounds. Jill has been here a week longer than I have and she's really starting to deal with some big problems. She says she almost wishes she was back in her first week detoxifying because that fog was a distraction. "Now I see everything too clearly," she says. Jill is in Blanche's group, so I don't know what her issues are. What goes on in group is supposed to be confidential, unless patients want to confide in each other. Jill's not the type to do that. She's one of the smilers, like me, always hiding behind her jokes.

3 P.M. I hate this new patient who came yesterday! He told the most disgusting joke at lunch about older women being like Australia: Everyone knows where Down Under is, but no one wants to go there. How dare he say that with older women in the room! I talked to Tony about it and he said, "So what did you tell him?" I said I couldn't confront him but maybe I will the next time when I've calmed down some. I know we're supposed to pay attention to the things in other people that get us upset because they may be our own defense mechanisms,

the very things we do or would want to do that we can't stand to look at in ourselves. I don't see how that applies in this case.

7 P.M. So I bite the bullet and call my husband and bring up this Australia joke. He says, "Why are you so upset? You don't even like sex." I tell him that's not true. I want to like it but I can't. Then I remember we're not supposed to say "I can't" and correct myself. I say, "I want to and I'm trying," but then I remember Vickie's "tryin' is lyin' " in that Southern accent of hers and get so frustrated. My husband is cool and intent on the other end of the phone, as if he's finally got my attention on something important to him. He says, "Maybe it's me." Then I really start to cry. "No, it's me," I say. "I'm just a fool." The truth is, how would I know? I've never slept with anyone but him, but I don't say that of course. He changes the subject and tells me Danny has moved back in for a while so he can catch a ride to work in the morning, and Kathleen is fine. She's dating a nice man who works in her office. That's a relief. I wish she would write or call me. I wish I were closer to my kids.

8 P.M. Jill and I do our laundry together. We talk about the Australia joke and my frustrating conversation with my husband. She says, "You're really upset about this so you should bring it to group." I tell her I can't do that. How can I talk about sex to Smitty with Tony and Mike in the room? She says if she's learned anything here it's that if I want to get better, the thing I don't want to do the most is the very thing I have to do. I think about that. Mike cried about how he doesn't have a sex life and wants one. He's very fat. I guess if he can make himself that vulnerable in front of women, I should be able to do it in front of men.

2 A.M. I wake up from a bad dream and start pacing the floor, then leave the room because I don't want to wake up my roommate. The lights are so bright around the nurses' station I go into the dining room. Slowly the dream comes into focus for me. I was lost, in an empty landscape, and no one in any direction to be found. It reminded me of a picture I saw once of the arctic tundra, stretching for miles and miles with nothing vertical any-

where to focus on, no landmarks of any kind, just emptiness, and for some reason it made me so sad. The dream was the same way, only instead of looking at the picture I was deep in the middle of it with that emptiness on every side.

I was crying so hard I didn't hear a nurse come in. She said, "We don't cry alone here." I apologized, and she put her arms around me. "Tell me why you're so upset," she said. "Did you have a bad dream?" I had to laugh. She sounded just like me with my kids when they were little. I told her and she said I was starting to get in touch with old feelings and not to be afraid. "You shut down a long time ago to protect yourself," she said, "but you're safe now. It's time you let these memories come out so you can live." I will never forget her.

5

Week Two

Came to Believe

Without a doubt, the first week of treatment is a disorienting time. The combined effects of withdrawal and the introduction of new ideas and behavior change cause most people to go into emotional overdrive. They don't know what they're feeling, but at least they're no longer numb and shut down. Of the three patients whose progress we are tracking through their journals, Jean is having the roughest time adjusting physically, from withdrawal of heavy caffeine, alcohol, and cocaine use. She had also been stressing her body with constant bingeing and purging with laxatives prior to treatment and her electrolytes were imbalanced. By the end of the first week, that condition has been righted, and she is now beginning to feel some complex emotions and erratic mood swings she hasn't had time to sort out because her concentration was on her physical discomforts.

Elaine, the compulsive overeater, has shown the most physical resilience, for her body responded immediately and gratefully to being fed at regular intervals. She, however, remains emotionally shut down and is relying heavily on her people-pleasing behavior to avoid the emptiness that is beginning to overwhelm her. Tony's physical condition has also improved, but his compulsion to control his stay (although on the surface he is friendly and compliant) is keeping him from making real progress.

It Is What You're Eating!

After seven days of following the food plan and abstaining from refined sugar, white flour, and caffeine, you must also be feeling quite differently about yourself. You may be noticing a diminishing of your obsession with food, particularly binge items, and a return of your morning appetite. Caffeine withdrawal rarely lasts more than a week, so you may already be enjoying the serenity and clearheadedness that comes after that drug has been flushed from your system.

You may also be noticing an improvement in your general mood. The empty feeling caused by bingeing, sugar, and caffeine may no longer be with you much of the time. Its lifting may be so gradual, and your acceptance of depression as your normal state so complete, that you may not even notice its absence for a while. You may be particularly aware of your new state of mind when you first wake up in the morning and in the late afternoon, when you were used to boosting your sagging mood with a jolt of caffeine and sugar. Your body is already thanking you even if your mind hasn't caught on to what you're doing yet.

In early abstinence, people often feel annoyed in the presence of those who do obsess about food. They, on the other hand, are not going to be happy about the decision you have made because it magnifies their problem. This is a difficult period, and the stress of being around people who are still bingeing may be too great. I suggest you avoid your eating buddies for a short time.

You Are a Celebration of Life

After saying your affirmations regularly for seven days, you will also be experiencing the first effects of positive self-talk. When you wake up in the morning, instead of the usual dread, you may be feeling a peaceful anticipation of the day. This is your subconscious mind at work, already processing the new messages it is so hungry to receive. Every now and then you may experience something someone once called a "s'mor," a "small moment of rapture." This feeling, brief though it may be, is a preview of the state of mind that is rightfully yours to own, the kind of feeling that should be constant merely for experiencing the miracle of being alive. When you feel a "s'mor," know your positive self-talk is beginning to work and that with continued practice, many more good feelings will follow. If you've rarely felt good about yourself, be prepared for the shock of it, and when it comes, don't reject it—rub it in! It's your birthright, no matter what kind of destructive messages you gave yourself in the past.

Meditation Is When You Listen

In the beginning, meditating is an act of will—willing the mind to settle, the body to quiet, controlling thoughts as they pass in and out of consciousness. With patient practice, that need to control disappears and the meditation process begins to work. Put your concentration on your breathing when the board meeting in your head is convened. Don't try to discourage all the cross-conversation, just blow it away with your breath. Orient yourself to your surroundings. Think of your feet as being conduits of energy from the ground that flows through your body and leaves through the top of your head. You are a receptor, listening for, not sending, messages. When those messages begin to be heard, they may be wordless. Sometimes they will take a visual form. Other times they will just be a feeling of quietude. You may not be aware of the answer when it fills your mind, only when you act on it. Suddenly you stop and say to yourself, "Why didn't I think of that before? How simple!"

In the beginning, you may be able to tolerate only a few minutes of meditation at a time. Don't worry about duration for now, just keep to a daily schedule and the time will extend itself.

You've Got to Move Your Body

One week of regular exercise is too brief a time for much to be happening to your body aside from some sore muscles, but you may assume that part of your new tranquillity is the result of the twenty to thirty minutes a day you are exercising. You may want to think about incorporating a new form of exercise into your daily routine, now that you have found how simple and pleasurable it is to make room for it, but remember, wherever you are and however busy you get, a half hour of brisk walking is always possible.

Hugs

If you're not making an effort to reach out to others, the changes you are making will be superficial and won't last. Because addiction is a disease of isolation, once you give up your love affair with a substance, your emptiness will drive you to despair unless you replace your loss with meaningful contact with the outside world. After a week of attending Anonymous meetings, you may already be feeling the urge to go up to newcomers and make them feel welcome. That urge is the healing message of this program already at work. The good that comes to you from it must be passed on in order for it to grow.

Other addicts readily understand the anguish of being alone while surrounded by people. Making the first move, establishing eye contact, and giving a hug sound so simple to accomplish, but to beginners still imprisoned in their isolation like you may have been just last week, breaking out is a seemingly impossible act of will. You know you're on the road to recovery when you first reach out to help someone else. If hugs don't come easy to you yet, or if you feel they are not always appropriate, try embracing with your eyes or a smile or the words "How are things going for you?" In the process, you will be infused with healing energy, an octane that will fill the uncomfortable void caused by the acknowledgment of your powerlessness. That power from without will fuel your recovery. You can't possibly experience it until you have shared or connected yourself to others. As long as we remain self-obsessed, it blocks our energy and makes it difficult to relate to others. All our lives we have been blaming our bodies for not getting the right mate, the promotion, or success on the playing field of life. As long as we scapegoated our bodies, we could avoid taking responsibility for our communications style and personalities. No addict wants to take responsibility, but it must be done.

Experience and express is the theme of the second week of treatment as we proceed on the path to intimacy. Acknowledging and moving through the pain of emptiness is essential to recovery. When you begin to tell yourself it is unendurable, think of it as childbirth. You are in a similar process, giving birth to your true nature, and there is no change without pain. I assure you it will pass.

Day Eight

TYPES OF COMMUNICATION

There are four basic types of communication: aggressive, passive, passive-aggressive, and assertive. Only assertive behavior truly communicates. The other forms rise out of hostility and fear, and they rarely work. Just because people use a particular behavior doesn't mean they *are* that behavior. They are free at any time to choose another style that will get them what they really want, but they have to discover what that behavior is before they can change it.

AGGRESSIVE

Aggressive types use threatening, accusing, fighting, and attacking behavior because they feel angry and frustrated. Much of the time they express themselves like little children, explosively, impulsively, and uncontrollably. They are demanding, dominating, and quick to blame and put down others. Rarely do they see themselves as aggressors. In fact, they often see themselves as victims! Unfortunately, their style of communication will only result in more anger and frustration, as others tend to dislike and avoid them. Aggressive people act under the misconception that they have the right to get what they want no matter the cost to someone else. They suffer from an "I" complex and see themselves as the center of the universe. The term "King Baby" often fits them perfectly. Their perception of the world is that someone has to win (themselves, of course) and someone else has to lose. Unless they are in the dominant position, they are so threatened they can't communicate, and their bottom line, "My way or the highway," makes compromise all but impossible.

It is difficult to get aggressive types to examine their behavior, and when they do see the truth about themselves, they are likely to respond with more anger and frustration because it is the only thing they know. Win-lose is their objective.

PASSIVE

Passive behavior is acting in a manner that allows other people to get what they want at the passive person's expense. Like the aggressive style, it is the behavior of little children: helpless, receptive, enduring what others impose without resistance. Whereas aggressors act like tyrannical two-year-olds, passive people act like infants. Their perception of the world is that somehow, somewhere, someone other than themselves will act responsibly and rescue them from the dilemma they're in.

A person who uses passive behavior quite naturally feels out of control and uses the behavior as an indirect way to control others. Underneath the placid surface is a lot of rage, and with the same lack of control that characterizes the behavior, the passive person will suddenly turn aggressive in a vain effort to regain control. The result is a lack of respect, from others and for oneself, and constant frustration. Passive people are an energy drain. People don't want to associate with victims, almost as if such behavior were contagious, and the passive person's inability to attract others only feeds into his or her feelings of worthlessness. Aggressives are full of contempt for their inability to take risks and seek them out for combat, for the passive person fits perfectly into their "I win–you lose" scenario.

PASSIVE-AGGRESSIVE

More common than either passive or aggressive behavior is a combination of the two. Because it appears to be adult behavior it is more socially acceptable. Passive-aggressive behavior is an indirect expression of hostility, resisting authority and controlling others, and it is much harder to detect, in oneself or in others, because it is childlike behavior in disguise. Anger and helplessness combine to take the form of clever sarcasm or unkind words, procrastination and dawdling, inefficiency or forgetfulness. Passive-aggressive types are the backstabbers, the ones who say, "Don't tell a soul but . . ." They are the ones who agree to do something and then come up with a last-minute excuse and leave you dangling. Devious and manipulating, they lose even when they win because they don't know whether they've won fair and square or because they've manipulated the results. Indirect to the extreme, they punish others by punishing themselves. Passive-aggressives like to seek out passive placators who don't think their ideas or feelings are worth defending, then walk all over them, hating the passivity they recognize, if not acknowledge, within themselves. They will also placate aggressive people and then seek to undermine them. I heard a definition recently from Robert Subby: Passive-aggressive is when a dog puts his paw on your shoulder, pisses on your leg, and licks your face at the same time!

ASSERTIVE

Whereas the other types of communication are defenses, often automatic in nature, that rarely get people what they want, assertiveness is a learned behavior that provides at the very least a feeling of respect if not the desired results. It's a general observation of mine that people will treat you with the same amount of respect as you command. No one ever gets it by pitiful pleading or an uproar. Only those whose behavior is a role model for respect will get it from others.

Assertive behavior is respectful of the rights of others. It is honest, direct, and firm. It makes self-expressive statements rather than asks questions. Assertive people think enough of themselves to express their thoughts and feelings without expecting others to agree with them. They have no need to control the responses of others, but they do need to be understood. They may not get what they want, but at least they're clear about what that is.

Nonassertive people confuse the goal of being liked with being respected. They have learned to act in inferior ways because they believe they *are* inferior, and that the rights of others are more important than their own. They are self-conscious before superior and authority figures. They are easily hurt by what others say and do. Their greatest fear is that they may offend. In their evasiveness, they often offend anyway, especially themselves, by constantly abnegating their own beliefs and desires and allowing others to maneuver them into situations they don't want to be in. To minimize their discomfort, they limit their experiences and don't use their full potential.

Assertive people respect themselves and others enough to tell the truth. They feel free to reveal themselves: "This is me. This is what I feel, think, and want." They can communicate with people on all levels—authority figures, strangers, friends, family, little children—with the same open, direct, honest, and appropriate manner. Their personalities do not change, chameleonlike, depending upon whom they are talking to. They enjoy the comfort that comes with simply being. They have an active orientation to life and go after what they want rather than what others tell them they should want. In contrast to the passive person who waits for things to happen, assertive people have the courage to go out and make things happen for themselves, and they enjoy the feeling of power that comes from growing up emotionally as well as intellectually, knowing they don't have to act like helpless children in order to get by in the world. Aware they can't always win, they gracefully accept their limitations and do not try to force their will on others. They strive in spite of the odds to make a good try, so whether they get their way or not, they maintain their self-respect. That's a win-win situation.

The difference between assertive and all other kinds of behavior is a combination of courage and respect. Aggressive people have no trouble finding the courage to say what's on their minds, but they lack respect for others. Passive people have too much respect for the opinion of others and lack the courage to express their own. Like the cowardly lion, the tin man, and the scarecrow in *The Wizard of Oz,* each type of communication lacks a quality that prevents a person practicing it from being whole and functioning.

Hardly anyone is assertive by nature, and it is a behavior rarely found in a person who grew up in a dysfunctional family where mixed messages were the norm. Assertive behavior is most often a learned skill. It is acting in a manner that allows a person to obtain what he or she wants while not violating the rights of others. That may seem like a tightrope act at first, but the insecurity will vanish with practice. Once you become comfortable in your new behavior, it will be infinitely better than the styles you have been using, which either allowed people to walk all over you or drove them away or made them confused, while it gave you feelings of discomfort that arise when you know you are not being true to yourself.

Imagine this situation: You are standing in a supermarket line and someone cuts in front of you. An aggressive person responds by making a scene—"How *dare* you!"—which often backfires. Others in line are offended more by the outburst than the original indiscretion and separate themselves from the aggressor. Sympathy may actually be generated for the trespasser because of the violence of the response. Passive people, on the other hand, are not fully convinced the offender doesn't have the right to usurp their place in line, and even if they do feel they have the right to protest, they are afraid to offend or ruffle feathers. Maintaining the peace is always their first objective. Meanwhile, they seethe inwardly, thinking of all the times they have felt helpless in the face of aggression.

Passive-aggressive people roll their eyes at others in line, murmuring under their breath about how "Some people have such nerve" and "Who do they think they are?" but never directly confront the offender. They may feel some relief in the approval of others but never justice, and their indirect form of communication, talking behind someone's back, is an indication to others that they can't be trusted.

The assertive person confronts the offender in a quiet but firm voice, using the "When you . . . I feel . . ." technique learned last week: "When you cut in line in front of me, I feel very angry." If the offender says, "So what? I don't care," assertive people are ready to plan a course of action and stick to it: "And if you don't go to the end of the line, I will talk to the manager." Assertive people don't need the support of others in the line, although they will often find they have their respect for being able to voice what the others may lack the courage to say, but winning a popularity contest is not the objective of the assertive person. Establishing and defending boundaries is. Even if the manager can't be found and the obnoxious line-cutter sails out of the supermarket without a reprimand, assertive people have the satisfaction of knowing they were true to themselves, worthy of protest. A lot of life's little inequities take place in situations similar to the supermarket line. People who fail to act assertively can put themselves into emotional tempests over these small infractions of the rules of good behavior, and their tranquillity can be disturbed for hours afterward. Because the infractions are minor and caused by strangers, such situations are a good place to practice assertive behavior. It's easier to confront a stranger than a significant person in your life, and each situation in which you act assertively—in spite of the fear and misgivings you feel—will give you the courage to change your behavior when it really counts.

Workbook for Day Eight

ASSIGNMENT ONE: YOUR HABITUAL COMMUNICATION STYLE

What is your habitual communication style: aggressive, passive, or passive-aggressive? Describe the last time you used it. Imagine you could go back to that moment. Describe how you could have responded assertively.

ASSIGNMENT TWO: "THE LIFE CHANGES SCALE"

The following is a helpful assessment tool called "The Life Changes Scale."* Completing and charting this scale will help you to better understand the underpinnings of your present communication patterns and how they have developed.

LIFE CHANGES SCALE

Please make one copy of this scale for each member of your family age 10 or older to complete. Each question means exactly what each family member perceives it to mean.

Write three answers in the space provided for each question.

In the blank to the left of each answer, write the number

*"The Life Changes Scale" was written by Tom M. Saunders, Ph.D. Dr. Saunders is a counseling psychologist in private practice in Winter Park, Florida. He is president and founder of The Chrysalis Foundation, Inc., which provides training in family systems throughout the country. This excerpt is reprinted by permission.

of the year that you would most associate with each answer.

When you have completed each answer with an associated year, follow the instructions at the end for charting your answers.

Name your three most intimate friends.

______ **1)** ____________________

______ **2)** ____________________

______ **3)** ____________________

Name your three most passionate enemies.

______ **4)** ____________________

______ **5)** ____________________

______ **6)** ____________________

Name your three most memorable incidents.

______ **7)** ____________________

______ **8)** ____________________

______ **9)** ____________________

Name your three illnesses of choice (what are your "target organs"?; to what does your body usually succumb?).

______ **10)** ____________________

______ **11)** ____________________

______ **12)** ____________________

Name your three most important personal issues under the category of "unfinished business."

________ 13) ______________________________

________ 14) ______________________________

________ 15) ______________________________

Name your three greatest losses.

________ 16) ______________________________

________ 17) ______________________________

________ 18) ______________________________

Name your three most significant geographical moves.

________ 19) ______________________________

________ 20) ______________________________

________ 21) ______________________________

Name your three greatest fears.

________ 22) ______________________________

________ 23) ______________________________

________ 24) ______________________________

Name your three favorite forms of dependency.

________ 25) ______________________________

________ 26) ______________________________

________ 27) ______________________________

Name your three best defenses (major life excuses used most often to avoid responsibility).

_______ 28) ___________________________________

_______ 29) ___________________________________

_______ 30) ___________________________________

INSTRUCTIONS FOR CHARTING:

Draw a scale using the model below as an example.

On the left end of the scale, print "BIRTH" and write your Month, Day, and Year of Birth.

On the right end of the scale, print "PRESENT" and write today's Month, Day, and Year.

Take each item # from the questionnaire, and place it on the scale. Use the Year which you assigned to each item # as a way of locating its relative position on the scale.

See the example below!

Month & Day of Birth					Today's Month & Day
____________					____________
	#2	#1	#3	#4	
BIRTH	______	______	______	______	**PRESENT**
Year of Birth	1	1	1	1	Today's Year
	9	9	9	9	
____________	4	5	6	8	____________
	7	6	4	4	

Name your three most intimate friends.

1956 1) Rhonda

1947 2) Christine

1964 3) Gerry

Name your three most passionate enemies.

1984 4) Marge

Tomorrow's workbook will show you how to interpret the results.

ASSIGNMENT THREE: HUGS

Have you established a schedule for attending Overeaters Anonymous meetings? Have you tried talking to people before they talk to you? Have you found it easier to give a hug than receive one? Is eye contact part of your hug?

HUGS

It's wondrous what a hug can do,
A hug can cheer you when you're blue.
A hug can say "I love you so,"
Or "Gee, I hate to see you go."
A hug is "Welcome back again,"
And "It's great to see you! Where've you
been?"
A hug can soothe a small child's pain
And bring a rainbow after rain.
The hug . . . there's just no doubt about it,
We scarcely could survive without it.
A hug delights and warms and charms,
It must be why God gave us arms.
Hugs are great for fathers and mothers,
Sweet for sisters, swell for brothers.
And chances are your favorite aunts
Love them more than potted plants.

Kittens crave them, puppies love them,
Heads of state are not above them.
A hug can break the language barrier,
And make your travels so much merrier.
No need to fret about your store of them,
The more you give the more there's more of
'em.
So stretch those arms without delay . . .
And give someone a hug today!

—AUTHOR UNKNOWN

A Day in the Life

JEAN

Monday. Have to write about yesterday because I played all day and didn't keep my journal. Tim, Miriam, this tiny anorexic, and I were giddy, chasing each other around like little kids, scaring each other and laughing. Tim carries Miriam upside down, running through the halls yelling, "Who wants a beefy anorexic?" and "I love the taste of stomach acid in the morning," another one of his bulimic jokes. He asks one of the nurses for an enema. The staff would say we are hiding our feelings, but I don't feel sad all the time. I need breaks. Then Tim, Chuck (this cute new guy), and I played Frisbee. Came back to a room full of people, Jill's family. She gets terribly nervous when her husband is here. She's real codependent and he's a recovering alcoholic. He tells her even the dog is depressed and won't eat now that she's here, and she forgets all about herself and has a codependent fit of worry and guilt. He sits here like a red-eyed lump, passively exuding misery. I want her to tell him to get lost, them, too—the fat daughter who cries, the fat son who stares at me as if I might explode—but the happy little baby can stay. I think Jill has to do it herself. I know she would resent it if I said anything. After all, I don't know what's good for her. I have plenty of other rooms to go in when they come in to mope.

This morning when I woke up, I felt the pang of that old betrayal to see my roommate's smoothly made bed. I know it's irrational and I would feel smothered if she woke me up, but I've been angry at other people all my life for not waking me up in the morning. I always feel like I've missed something. I know it's my responsibility, but I never even hear the nurse when she comes in to wake us. My insomnia kicks in at midnight. I was deeply asleep last night and it woke me up so I could lie awake and think disturbing thoughts about nothing. Now I'm groggy.

We get weighed. I've gained two pounds. They're sitting on my stomach like a little pillow. Oh, well. At least my head is clear and my food stays down. Haven't even thought about wanting to bring it up for a few days. It's funny how little I've been thinking of food at all. Mostly I've been thinking about Tim and a couple of the other men here. I know I should accept the fact that it's inappropriate to sleep with people here and to always be the center of attention. People are here to work on themselves, and they can help me but they don't have to. I guess I have to bring this up in group. All my attractions do is take the focus off myself where I need it the most. I will use them as a signal to bond platonically without the power games of sex. Or at least try to do that. I wonder if I can.

9:30 A.M. I told Danny, this heavy, older man who's leaving, that when he made sexual jokes about me I felt self-conscious and he agreed not to. Things feel easier between us now. I can look into his eyes.

12:30 P.M. I can't believe how fantastic I feel. Father Booth was here this morning. He talked about spirituality, which would normally put me right to sleep because of my boring minister father. But Father Booth says spirituality is not the same as religion. He says it's about being a positive and creative human being. You don't have to "get spirituality" like people "get religion" because we already have it. It's just covered over with the negativity and self-destruction that led us into addiction. He draws a square with a dot in the center and asks everyone what they see. We say, "A dot." He says, "Don't look at the dot. Look at the space around it." The dot is like criticism. It's just a tiny pinpoint, but it becomes the focus if you let it. He tells us being positive and creative means working your buns off. If we keep hiding who we are, we'll stay the same. We can't get better if we're sitting on a secret or if we're controlling the program.

Afterward I hugged him real hard and he looked at me and said, "Go for it!" I feel more purposeful and positive. I'm having fun with other people. I feel loved and like I can be myself. I feel better about everything. I really do. Father Booth is so smart, it's subversive. Subversive to depression, I mean.

I'm sorry I wrote so nastily about Blanche, my counselor. I don't feel so critical of her today. I think I was jealous of her self-assuredness the other day, but now that mine is returning, she doesn't bother me.

1 P.M. Group therapy. Blanche was talking about the similarities between the obese and the anorexic patients. She had some people change chairs so we were on opposite sides of the room. Danny made a joke about the room starting to tilt. Similarities—they're both uncomfortable. Anorexics have to sit on their bones. Overeaters can't go to the bathroom on planes, have to ask for seatbelt extensions. Both obsess on food, make a relationship out of it. Both don't like the way they look, think they're too fat and worry about gaining weight. Obese patients are addicted to eating, the anorexics to not eating. Then she asked Charlene, this terribly thin girl, what she weighed. She said in her tiny voice, "Ninety-three pounds," and Danny says, "My *leg* weighs ninety-three pounds." Everyone but Charlene thought that was pretty funny. When Danny isn't being sexist, he does have a good sense of humor. Then Miriam told on Charlene, said she was exercising secretly in her room and wearing leg weights under her jeans and was the last one to leave the dining room so no one would see she didn't eat her food.

Then other people in the group started in on Charlene, how she isolates in her room, doesn't know people's names, wanted to know why she didn't speak more in group, why she didn't raise her voice so people could hear her. Finally Gloria, angry Gloria who never has a good thing to say about anybody or anything, started to cry. "Leave her alone," she said. "She's a good kid." Gloria is all of nineteen herself. I spoke up them and said I was really surprised, because I didn't think Gloria cared about anybody, and Gloria glared at me and flung her hair the way she does.

Blanche told Charlene that getting well was entirely up to her. They couldn't help her if she didn't want to live. She said anorexics had the hardest time getting better because they were so good at controlling, and that starving yourself was a painful way to die. All this time Charlene didn't say a thing. I kept looking at her as she stared off into space and a shudder went through me. I had to blink my eyes to keep her in focus, as if she were fading away. She's so pretty, or was. Now she looks like an old woman—her nose is beaked, her chin is sharp. She got very pinched looking when Blanche was talking about her not wanting to live. A chill went through me as I watched her because I'm afraid she's going to die. I'm afraid of the anorexics. I know I'd be one if I had their control, but I keep hearing how I'm out of control, erratic. I know that's true, but don't know why or what to do about it.

3 P.M. We saw a video in Wellness that got me all upset. It's called *The Silent Scream* and shows all these kids talking about how they'd been sexually abused. This one little girl really got to me, her face so sweet and open, her big wide eyes, talking about how she had been molested by her mother's boyfriend. I got so upset I had to leave the room. Blanche came looking for me and found me lying on my bed. I didn't know what to say. She kept asking me what the film had brought up, why I couldn't stay in the group, and I told her I didn't want to talk about it. Maybe later. I just felt so sorry for that little kid.

Then Tim and Debbie came into my room. They wanted to know if I was all right. I started to cry and said I just felt so sorry for those little kids, those innocent faces. Debbie told me she was molested by her uncle and I told her I was sorry for her, too, but I didn't want to hear about it. Then Tim jumped up and said, "Let's go feed the ducks," so we did. But I couldn't stop seeing that little kid's face in front of me.

9:30 P.M. Went to an AA meeting tonight and it was good. I'm eight days clean. It's a really big meeting, lots of laughter, cigarette smoking, and coffee drinking. Of course those of us from Janet Greeson's "A Place For Us" pass up the coffee unless there's a decaf urn and are very virtuous about not eating the cookies. On Mondays people come up and get anniversary poker chips of different colors, and there was a long line for Day One. I suppose people give up drinking and drugging after a weekend bender, like me. I feel like an old-timer with eight days. We broke up into small groups and I shared. I don't even remember what I was talking about, but all of a sudden I started to cry. People around the table were understanding. Finally I just said, "I can't talk," and the woman next to me stroked my arm. "It gets better," she said. That made me cry more. Why is it that when people acknowledge my pain instead of trying to talk me out of it, I get even more emotional? Where are all these tears coming from? They feel thick and old.

10 P.M. I called my sister. I don't know why I got the urge, and wish I hadn't. She was surprised to hear from me. We had our usual superficial conversation. Right before she hung up (I could hear her husband in the background calling to her in that demanding voice of his, just like Dad's) she said, "Are you all right, Jeanie?" "No," I said. "I'm not all right. That's why I'm here." Then she got off the phone real fast. I felt so all alone, like there was no one in the world to protect me. Then I got this sudden desire to see Gloria. Wouldn't dare presume to knock on her door and ask to see her, so I knocked on her door and asked if Elaine was there. She was on the phone and Gloria just glared at me with this "What do you want?" look on her face, so I just left.

Day Nine

INTERPRETING "THE LIFE CHANGES SCALE"

How You Respond

As you have recently learned, one of *your* rights is to be responsible for how you perceive and report an experience. There are no hidden meanings in "The Life Changes

Scale." The results are today's snapshot of how you view your life to date, and what it means to you now. If you would like to discover where your important changes fit with those of your family members, you may wish to copy this scale and give it to the important members of your family network to complete, then compare results with them at a later time.

As you recall, the instructions reminded you, "Each question means exactly what each family member perceives it to mean." Some of the descriptors may seem a little strange at first. Perhaps you have never considered "passionate" as an adjective for "enemies." But passionate is a good synonym for "intense," and generally, when we are busy assigning those feelings which we do not wish to own as the property of another, we become passionately involved in that process of blaming.

"Illnesses of *choice*" is another uncommon phrase. Few would acknowledge ever electing illness, yet none would deny that the daily stress, fatigue, and improper nourishment with which we punish our physical body must undermine the immune system, and handicap it at best.

The "Year" assigned in the blank to the left of each numbered item is a "best guess" as to the year that we associate with that item becoming important in our lives. Again, being exact is not important.

As always, your conscious judgmental mind has done its best to interfere with your response to each item. For those persons who have learned to be afraid of being responsible for their "Rights," the words of cartoon character Pogo could not be more correct: "We have met the enemy, and they is us!" For this reason, you may want to wait a few days, and then complete "The Life Changes Scale" a second time; the results will be quite different if you follow your heart, and respond in writing to the first flash of a response that comes to your mind.

Charting the Results

Draw a scale like the one in the example, but allow yourself more room. On the left end of the scale is the date of *your birth*, perhaps the most important day of your life! At the right end of the scale is today's date, the second most important day of your life.

Commencing with item #1 and the Year assigned to that item, estimate approximately where that year would fall on the scale between your birth year and now. Write the year just below the scale, as shown in the example, and the corresponding item number just above the scale. Continue, in the same manner, with each item until all thirty items have been charted.

Discovering the Clusters

As you review the results of your charting, you will notice that *changes* usually do not happen in "ones." Changes will usually occur in groups.

Circle any Year or Years that have two or more items assigned to them. As you remember that year, at this moment, try to recall any other significant changes that happened during that same approximate time span.

For those of you who have asked other family members to complete this exercise, when they have finished all of the above, compare notes with them. Do any of your significant years of change correspond with theirs? It will be helpful to hear their perceptions of what was happening during those important years as well. In this way, you will begin to better understand the significant events in your life as well as the backdrop against which they happened.

Just as in the solar system or the atom, each particle is in delicate balance with every other particle. No one family member ever goes through a transition that does not in some way affect every other family member in the system.

What Does It All Mean?

"The Life Changes Scale" was first developed in 1987 as a research tool for The Chrysalis Foundation, Inc., of Winter Park, Florida. Chrysalis' President/Founder, Tom M. Saunders, Ph.D., has worked with families for over twenty years, and currently maintains a private practice in Florida called Family Systems Consultants.

Through the years, Dr. Saunders had observed that

when family members were seen individually and made excellent progress over a period of time, their progress was often limited by the onset of other problems in the family. A teenager who had been acting out, now back on a positive track, was followed into treatment by a depressed mother. By the time the mother had harnessed her creativity and was actively pursuing a more fulfilling life, her husband would have a heart attack, thereby forcing the oldest child to return home from college to help support the family.

At first, these "coincidences" were discarded as projections of the therapist, and ignored. However, when the same patterns were observed over a period of years in one family after another, interested colleagues began to join Dr. Saunders in the research effort.

Of all their findings the most fascinating is perhaps the "ethernet phenomenon." Remember the bump-um cars at the county fair? Those cars were powered by electricity through a pole at the rear of the car that reached to touch an electrical net about eight feet overhead. When one car would strike another hard enough to jar it off the net, the car would not be operational until it was pushed into place again, touching the net once again.

Families appear to be connected by such an energy net—a sixth sense, an unconscious, spiritual electrical field through which all important communication takes place. Through work with both Chrysalis and Family Systems Consultants, Dr. Saunders has discovered that family members, though separated by geographical boundaries, emotional isolation, and no physical communication, still experience their major clusters of changes during the same periods of time, plus or minus six months. Even those families who have not spoken for periods of twenty years or more will encounter the same changes, just as if there had been an ongoing dialogue.

It is interesting to note that most people do not believe in this familial connection when they first hear about it. Yet those same individuals are quick to acknowledge that all animals and probably most children have such sixth-sense information available. Few, regardless of their scientific persuasions, would try to fool a Doberman or horse of whom they were afraid.

The Meaning of Change

Change is healthy. Change is necessary. Change must involve dying and being reborn. Change, by definition, means taking a new risk and being responsible for the consequences.

However, as alluded to earlier, individual change never happens in a vacuum. When one member of a family risks doing anything substantially different, the entire family system must begin to adjust, ever so slightly, to accommodate that new change.

The most natural reaction of any family system, however, is to try to maintain "status quo" at any cost! The family will almost always try, at an unconscious level, to pull the changing member back into his or her old behavior even though the support of the family is critical if that change is to remain for any length of time.

A parallel phenomenon exists in the overnight religious conversion. Swept up in a powerful emotional tidal wave, these individuals, surrounded by enormous love and support, make a decision to change their way of living in favor of gaining more of this support from others. However, when they return home, their family and friends still see them as they were and treat them as they always have. Any positive change, because of the powerful pull of the family, becomes difficult to maintain.

Enslavement or Isolation

Part of the value of identifying these personal and family changes is that it allows us to better understand the impact which these changes have had upon the individual and the system of which he or she is a part. Losing weight, as an example, has far greater impact than those shed pounds. It means giving up an entire role, a place in the sun, if you will—a direct link to a special relationship to at least one member of the family, and usually several others.

Liz's story is a good example. Her mother has been tracking her weight since Liz was in junior high. With the same zeal as the spouse of an alcoholic who counts drinks and bottles, Mom has always been chiding Liz about how much she eats, how little she eats, how many diets she has tried, and so on. Yet, any substantial loss of weight has always been put down with sarcasm.

Liz's father doesn't say much. He began to touch Liz inappropriately just about the same time that Liz began to obsess about weight. Liz has avoided her father ever since and has never told Mom because it could mean that her parents' underground Cold War could become a divorce. To make matters worse, Liz's brother, five years her senior, came home quite drunk one evening, accidentally got into bed with Liz, and blacked out.

Liz has "swallowed" everything and kept the family secrets intact. However, the sad implication of her losing her weight is that she fears losing both her parents, their marriage, and her older brother at the same time.

While not all family dynamics are as tragic, the implication of enslavement or isolation is a part of every family. If we do whatever seems necessary to save our family and keep them intact, we become enmeshed with them to a point of losing our own identity. At the other extreme, if we attempt to take care of our own needs, we risk isolation.

Who we are, and how we are, is always a part of this ongoing paradox. Our level of assertive communication relates directly, at any given moment, to where we are in this process of separating ourselves from our original family system. Ironically, wherever we happen to become stuck in this process is the role that we continue to play and replay in every social system of which we become a part, including marriage.

A Change of Role, a Change in Communication

What must become obvious by now is that how we communicate is a direct representation of the role which we have elected to play in our family, our work life, our social setting, and our marriage. Don't ever be fooled by passive persons telling you that they have no power, but truly wish for some. When passive persons can't decide where they would like to eat, either someone will rise to the occasion to make the decision for them, feed them, or leave them to their own devices to starve to death. Most passive people get fed.

If you have trouble believing in the "ethernet" concept, think about how all of these matched pairs in the world find each other.

For the aggressive person who likes to bulldoze and run other people's lives, there are always others available who just can't wait to be told what to do, all the while complaining bitterly about their lot in life. However, the best part of having your life run for you is that there is only a minimal level of responsibility to meet, such as hygiene, tying your shoes, and the like.

The change-up artist, the passive-aggressive, obviously needs to be matched with someone adequately skilled to do the same intricate dance. These individuals are usually more exciting since they play many roles, of either variety, and can turn on a dime, if necessary, to change directions. The bad news is that when you have seen their performance, it's time to move on to another relationship.

To be assertive is to risk change. Like most quality spices, a little goes a long way. One of the early faults of assertiveness training was that the newly skilled pledges would leave their classrooms, rear their heads, and assert all over anyone around them in the name of changing their role. For the unsuspecting spouse or friends, this often meant the death of a relationship because the newly assertive person had never bothered to understand the power of the unresolved anger cooking just below the surface.

Striking a match creates power and energy. Fueling that spark with gasoline makes a powerful combination. But it takes a great deal of practice to control just the right amount of spark and mix it with the right amount of gasoline to attain the right amount of energy needed for the occasion.

Permanent Change Is Gradual

It was a high school physics teacher who taught me this valuable lesson about sparks and gasoline. He pointed out that since gasoline contains no oxygen, a flame cannot burn without the right amount of air. He would put one drop of gasoline in a Coke bottle, and hold a lit match to the top of the bottle. Nothing. Not until the bottle contained three drops of gas would a blue flame shoot from the top. Nor would four or five drops do the trick. Just the right amount of air and the right amount of gas . . . with a spark . . . produce the right amount of flame.

Changing roles is just as gradual. Just like changing a golf or tennis swing, it takes a great deal of practice to program the brain. Changing roles takes risking a new role time and time again until it begins to become familiar.

An old vaudeville joke makes the point. A gentleman in a hurry asks a New York cab driver to pull over to the curb where he inquires through the window, to a policeman on the corner, "How do I get to Carnegie Hall?" The policeman replies, "Practice, practice, practice!"

It was the French philosopher and scientist Pascal who wrote one of the most interesting things I've read about God. Pascal hedged his bet by saying that not believing in God had no consequences if there were no God. But if there were a God, he continued to reason, then everything would be in favor of being a believer. And it is belief in God that makes the change in behavior necessary.

Pascal said that at the point of confessing to believe in God, the new believer must act *as if* there is a God. One must pray *as if* prayer will be answered, kneel *as if* one is humble, and in doing so, obtain faith.

Permanent change is accomplished in just such tiny steps. Each day, each hour, each moment, must be lived *as if* the responsible change is possible, *and in that moment, change occurs!*

A Day in the Life

TONY

9:30 A.M. I got the word I'm not to make any more business calls. My medical reports are not good, the doctors say. My blood pressure is too high, cholesterol, glucose, and triglyceride levels out of sight, and I'm generally stressed out. At least I've dropped eight pounds. Everything else has stayed the same, and they say it's because I'm not really giving myself a chance to get better when I'm focused on the outside all the time. I tell them I can't do what they ask. My business will fall apart, and they tell me either I give it a try for a few days or they will discharge me. They're serious. I think about it for a while. Maybe it's no accident that this morning when I was getting yet another round of blood tests the nurse ran out of my room when she heard a voice on the loudspeaker call, "Code Blue. ICU Ten." I knew that meant someone was in a life-and-death situation down in the cardiac unit. So I told the counselor I'd try it for a few days.

"And limit your personal calls to evenings," the counselor said. I got a little miffed at that, but I guess I am too wound up in everyone's problems. I could use the break.

11 A.M. I have an individual session with Smitty. He wants to know when I'm going to start working in group. I tell him I just don't have anything serious to bring up. I wasn't abused or anything as a kid. He said, "You don't have to go all the way back to the past. How about your wife's illness? How about your problems with your brother, or your son? Those are all issues you could talk about in group. Or maybe there isn't anything that's bothering you."

Well, I know that's not true. I told him I'm new to all this, and I'm not used to making myself vulnerable. He asked me how I felt about the others when they let down their guard and really got honest. I said I felt closer to them, admired them for it. "So what have you got to lose?" Smitty said. He's right, I know, and I like him a lot. I guess I'd better get down to work. Now that I've unpacked and all!

1 P.M. I was going to open up in group, but it was Mike's turn to spill and he really went at it. He's so angry that he's wasted all this time here being a good guy and now he's just got a few days to go and he feels he hasn't really gotten to what's bothering him. So much control, capped tight by his intellect and his intense need to be there for everyone. He starts yelling at himself for being so caught up in being liked, being everyone's father confessor, and pretty soon he's not yelling at himself but at

someone else. Smitty asks him who he's mad at and he says, "Everyone." But Smitty won't let him get by with that. Pretty soon this big, soft, kindly man is beating his fists on a pillow, angry at priests and nuns and a grandfather who humiliated him, a father who deserted him, brothers and sisters who didn't care. He's roaring with anger. I couldn't believe there was so much anger in the guy. Elaine is practically out the door, and Leslie, a new patient who just came in yesterday, looks like she's about to follow. After Mike was through being angry, Elaine started complaining about her roommate and the towels she leaves on the bathroom floor, and then the new person says she's gay and someone made a homophobic comment and she doesn't feel she can open up here and is afraid she's come to the wrong place. There were too many problems on the table. I didn't feel right about adding my own.

10 P.M. Called the wife and told her about my new restrictions. She laughed. She said, "What's that going to do to a workaholic? What are you going to take up to fill the gap?" I told her I'd have to live with it. It's like all we ever do is joke. The things I'd really like to ask her, like what's really on her mind, is she scared about her cancer coming back, all the things I know she lives with, I can't somehow. All these things are off limits. I miss her. I wish I could tell her that, too, but I'm afraid she'll take it as just another burden to carry.

Day Ten

SELF-IMAGE: IF I AM NOT MY BODY, THEN WHO AM I?

In the first week of treatment, the behavior patterns that people use to protect themselves are identified. In the second week they are shaken loose and, if the patient is secure enough, discarded. In the absence of these protective behaviors, often developed early in life, patients feel temporarily helpless, unshielded, and vulnerable.

No one is likely to take such a risk except in the safe environment a treatment center or individual or group therapy offers. If you were unable to identify any of your defense mechanisms last week, you are a likely candidate for therapy. Today I will reiterate those defenses, plus a few more, as they apply to the three patients, Jean, Elaine, and Tony, in their progress so far. In this way, you may be able to take another look at what it is you're doing that's keeping you stuck. This week the three patients will begin to identify the behavior patterns they are using. Other people, whom they are coming to trust, will point out those behaviors and convince them that what they think is protecting them is actually hindering their development.

Like most people, you may find it easier to identify these characteristics in others than see them in yourselves. As you read, whatever evokes emotions, especially strong feelings of negativity, is the clue to look for your own participation in these behavior patterns. Self-discovery is difficult, for defense mechanisms become as familiar and cherished as old shoes. I want you to look for the nail in those shoes, the pain which we ignore or do not tend to. That pain may seem to be coming from somewhere else—your job, disappointing relationships, bad luck, fate—but willingness to search for the real source will be the only way to stop the hurting.

Under stress Jean, the bulimic, acts aggressively, although it is difficult for her to see her behavior as anything other than defensive. In group interactions her behavior patterns are becoming clear to others if not to herself.

BLAMING

Jean sees her problems as being caused by her jealous and emotionally unstable mother, her dominating and manipulative father, her competitive and people-pleasing sister, and her abusive ex-husband. She is so preoccupied with their faults she can gloss over her own contributions to the endless conflicts in her life. By constantly *creating crisis* she gets lost in the details of the chaos, which protects her from having to look at what's really going on.

IMPULSIVENESS

Jean's impulsiveness drives her from one end of the emotional spectrum to the other. Her moods change from one moment to the next, as well as her opinions of others. Her *promiscuity* is another defense. She relates to others sexually rather than as people as a way of *avoiding intimacy*, which frightens her.

ENMESHING

All her life Jean has been unsure about where she ends and other people begin. Her enmeshment with her family, constantly playing the role assigned to her of Bad Girl, at the same time she tries to win their approval, contributes to her lack of identity. Already she is involved in a popularity contest among the younger patients and is becoming the spokesperson for others who want to confront Gloria about her antisocial behavior. Jean impulsively takes on the role of chief confronter because it is what she has always done.

ANALYZING DATA

Jean loves to try to make sense of what's happening, but experience and understanding can't happen simultaneously. In order to experience she would just have to be, and that is too threatening for Jean to attempt at this point. Analysis keeps her in her head and her body at bay.

PERFORMING

Because she is so bright and so verbal, people are drawn to her. Her *extremism* and well-developed *humor* make for good storytelling, but they mask what's really happening. Jean's need to be "on," the center of attention, keeps her out of touch with her real feelings.

REBELLION

If Jean can redirect the energy she puts into her combativeness, she will be able to make great strides. For the moment, she doesn't feel safe enough to drop her defenses as a warrior against injustice and fight her addiction instead. She needs to feel safe to do that, and having never felt that way, she doesn't trust the loving environment she has found herself in. But she wants to. Her lack of passivity is her saving grace.

PEOPLE-PLEASING

Elaine's major defense mechanism is to keep everybody happy, but no matter how hard she tries, she fails. Her efforts to get close to people like Jean don't succeed because they see her as a phony. She is able to get close only to other people-pleasers, and the intimacy of that contact is shallow because they all have the same objective—to be liked rather than to get to know each other.

CARETAKING

By the third day in treatment, Elaine had taken a new patient under her wing. She is constantly on the alert for ways to meet others' needs, and the question she asks most is, "Is there anything I can do?" Her caretaking extends to her husband and daughter at home. She worries that they won't be able to function without her, then gets upset when they can.

BEING NONDIRECT

Elaine is a classic passive-aggressive. She lacks the courage to be confrontive, particularly with her formidable roommate Gloria, and so she gets involved indirectly in other people's affairs. *Piggybacking* is one of the ways she becomes involved, identifying with others who do take action as long as doing so doesn't interfere with her people-pleasing. Her *busyness* keeps her mind off her problems, particularly her family life, which is in a shambles.

Her concentration on whether other patients are abiding by the rules and whether she should tell on them fills up her emptiness. *Smiling* keeps others at bay, *forgetting* her home situation makes it easier to smile, and by *numbing her body* she hopes to keep old, fearful feelings from rising.

Although Elaine is full of defenses, she truly wants to find a way out of the dilemma she's in. She desires the peace of mind she has never known, and she is willing to look at her behavior and see it for what it really is, even if it disgusts her.

DENIAL

Tony, on the other hand, is not willing to look. Of the three patients, he has made the least progress and is still in deep denial. Denial is a way people learn to live in a hostile environment, and Tony's work and family life is certainly that. Although Tony is well liked by the other patients, emotionally he is *isolating.* Although he has big problems, he is constantly *minimizing* them. In group therapy he is *playing safe,* and surprisingly *compliant* for someone who is so aggressive in his professional life. He has learned how to avoid conflict when he doesn't have to confront.

In treatment, we work hard at challenging defense structures because you can't bond when you're defensive. Imagine two medieval knights in full armor embracing each other, giving each other's helmet a peck. That's how close you can get when you haven't let go of your defense mechanisms.

During this second week, as the self-image begins to crack, patients need to look to others to see how they are doing, for they are still convinced the image they have been portraying is their real self. They believe they are who they are by what they have achieved, the roles they play in life of wife, husband, son, daughter, student, employee. How others see them is the only confirmation they feel they have, particularly at a time when they are not sure whether the image they have been projecting is really how the world has seen them after all. In such an insecure time, they find it necessary to hide the feelings, wants, and needs of their real selves, for that identity is still too nebulous to hold on to. Instead, they become intensely involved with how others see them, as if they would disappear without that reference. They are particularly attracted to other addicts, who also believe in the "I am not enough" dictum. With all the deprivations they have been going through—of food and other mood-altering substances, plus their inability to practice their workaholism and relationship addictions—they are intensely devoted to externals.

Inside, the person they really are still feels like a void. They feel empty, fragmented, full of rage and hurt like little children abandoned by their parents in a room without toys, deprived, helpless, and confused. When they are not feeling the anger and pain of loss of identity, they feel an abyss of nothingness. They are bored, listless, distracted, depressed.

If you feel the same way, rejoice. This stage, painful though it may be, is part of a process you are now engaged in. If you don't allow these feelings to be experienced and expressed, they will intensify to the point where you will have to numb them with food or another substance, creating a little short-term pleasure for some more long-term pain, and then you'll be back on the roller coaster again, hating all the "downs." If you allow yourself to experience and express these feelings, they will be done with and you can move on. Your need for help at this point may be overwhelming. Tomorrow we will discuss what to look for in a therapist.

If you are not experiencing any feelings, either you don't have an addiction to food or you're kidding yourself. That's just another defense. It may work for a while, but the real you knows better. Keep reading, and remember the people who are in the most pain are the ones who are numb. Perhaps you should be asking yourself what your numbness is concealing. What could be the source of this pain of yours that is so great you have to shut down all feelings?

Moving from external to internal is a process that involves developing a healthy body image, exercise and good nutrition, boundary development, reality testing, and taking action. By avoiding the comparison of yourself to others, striving for balance and less rigidity, and realizing that perfectionism never leads to happiness, you can keep committed to this process. It doesn't happen by magic or overnight, the way we addicts like it, but it does happen.

Workbook for Day Ten

ASSIGNMENT ONE

Go back to week one, day one, and look over the list of defense mechanisms again. See if you can find some you use that you didn't acknowledge last week.

ASSIGNMENT TWO

Describe three experiences you have had since last week in which you were aware of using a defensive behavior pattern. What was the reason for your needing to protect yourself? What was the result? Did it get you what you wanted?

You Are a Celebration of Life

To the affirmation of the first week, add this additional line:

I am not my body.
I am free.
I am as God created me.
I am part of a community.

A Day in the Life

ELAINE

Wednesday. I'm so thrilled I've lost six pounds. I've managed to lose that much in a week before, but only by feeling terribly deprived. The food here satisfies me, and eating regularly makes me feel like I'm really taking good care of my body. In gratitude, my body is happy. There's a spring to my step when I go for my walk. My roommate has all these bottles of lotions and oils in the bathroom, and I've been using the all-over bath oil after my shower. I really scrub my feet and lower legs. They've been so rough and scaly for years, and I just don't take the time to really work on them on a day-to-day basis. I spend a few extra minutes in the shower scrubbing off dead skin and then steal some of my roommate's bath oil. I'll buy some for myself this weekend.

11 A.M. I have a one-on-one with Smitty. He wants to know what's going on with me, when I'm really going to get down to business. I tell him he really makes me nervous. Finally he gets out of me this problem I have not wanting to have sex with my husband, particularly since the affair he had with the younger woman. He asks me to ask him to come down for family therapy next week. I get really upset about that. Am I that sick? He says family therapy would be very healing in our case. How about my son and daughter? Was there a chance they could come, too? I told him I didn't think so, but I'd ask. He wants me to start talking in group about my family problems, with my husband and my children. I tell him I will, but it's so hard for me to talk about sex with these men! How I wish I had Blanche or Vickie for group.

1 P.M. Tony really talked in group for the first time, about his brother. Says he's trying to undermine Tony in the family business. Tony wants to check out and go home to take care of this crisis he has that came up this morning, and then come back. Smitty keeps asking him about what his problem is with his brother from way back so Tony won't go on and on talking about this business deal and that business deal, but Tony's real tough to distract and keeps interrupting. His face gets red and his veins stick out. Then in a rush comes this story about how he's the oldest but his brother has always been the favorite, better in school, at sports, with women, but a bit of a prodigal son while Tony has had to take responsibilities—his sisters, aunts, cousin, mother, father—they all look to Tony to make things fair and then get mad at him when they don't like the outcome.

Smitty asks the group what they think. There's silence at first because everyone's sort of afraid, although respectful, of Tony. He's a powerful person in the group and plays the same role here as he does on the outside. Finally I say, "Do you really have to be the one to solve all the problems—or do you want to be?" He sort of laughs at that. "Maybe a little of both," he says. Then Mary says, "Why don't you take it easy? Maybe while you're here they'll have to find a way to settle their own disputes." Smitty talks about his need to control everyone and everything. Tony says he doesn't see how that could be so because at the moment everything in his life is out of control. Smitty tells him to write a letter to his brother and read it to the group.

I was relieved when Tony went on and on about his problem, but when he was finished, I took a deep breath and brought up the joke Tom the family therapist told that offended me so, and I practiced confronting him: "When you told me the joke about the older women and their sexuality, you offended every woman in the room." The group really jumped down my throat and told me to speak for myself. I tried again. "When you told that joke, I felt humiliated." I got so angry when I said that! I almost blacked out. I could hear Smitty's voice from far away. "How did you feel humiliated?"

"I didn't deserve that," I said. "It really hurt."

Smitty said, "Do you hear what's happening to her voice?"

Tony said, "Like a little girl."

"It's not fair!" I wailed.

"Don't look down and cover your eyes," said Smitty. "That's about shame. What's not fair?"

"To ridicule me like that, my body. How dare you make fun of me!"

"Who are you talking about, Elaine? Who's this little girl inside you talking about?"

And then the words "My father" ripped out of my throat, from a place so deep inside me I had never felt it before. Old tears came up out of my throat like phlegm.

"Open your eyes, Elaine." Smitty's voice was still

from far away. "What did your father say that humiliated you?"

"I just had my bath. I was running around, dancing, without any clothes on. Just this little baby. And he took a broom—"

The memory that had flashed in my mind like an old movie was in full Technicolor. Now it flickered. The screen went blank.

"I don't remember," I cried.

"Your father's dead now. He can't hurt you. You're safe here. This is the place to talk about what happened. Bring it back. What did he do with the broom?"

"He just hit me with it, because I was so naughty, running around and showing off my body. He hit me and told me I was bad."

I could feel the sharpness of that pain, and the fall to the floor. I could hear the angry, righteous voice of a man who had died when I was too young to remember. Now this was the only memory I had of him and that was too painful to bear. "I made it up," I said. "It never happened."

"Do you think Elaine's making this up? Is this a performance on her part?" said Smitty. People's voices floated out to me like a caress. "It's real, Elaine." "We believe you, Elaine." "Stay with it, Elaine."

"Look around the room at the faces. What do you see?"

I looked. I was crying so hard the faces seemed to be underwater: at comforting Mary, whose lap I had a great urge to crawl into, at Tony with tears in his eyes, at Kathryn, who was openly weeping, for herself, too, maybe, at wisecracker Tim sitting solemnly next to me with his arm around my chair, at the new patient, Leslie, looking scared and withdrawn but obviously convinced that what she was witnessing was no performance on my part. "Love is what I see," I said.

"Where's your mother?" said Smitty. A roar came out of me then. "Right there!" I said. "Doing nothing. Agreeing with him that I was a bad girl. Oh, what's happening to me? Where are these awful feelings coming from?"

"They're coming up now because it's safe to remember here," said Smitty. "Ask the group if it's bad for a little baby to want to dance naked around the room after her bath, a cute little baby who feels good without her clothes on."

"He had no right to hit you for that," said Tony.

"You were innocent," said Tim. "Innocent then, innocent now."

The group ended the way it always does, standing in a tight circle breathing into the Serenity Prayer. I hung on to the words for dear life. Afterward no one moved from the circle for a minute, feeling the closeness. Then arms were cradling me from every direction and I was encompassed by unconditional love. I felt transported by that love, floating on it. I could bear up. No one had ever known what I had just revealed, for I had been too ashamed even to remember it, and what had mattered so much all these years just didn't matter anymore. I couldn't change the fact that it had happened, but I could change what it had done to me, the attitude I had about my body, how my whole life no one had ever seen me naked, how I had begun at an early age to eat to conceal that little naked body, enveloping it in layer upon layer of fat, assuring it would be covered up, never looking at it except stealthily or accidentally, in parts but never whole, too painful to see whole. Suddenly I loved this body of mine that had been shamed by two people who didn't know better, didn't know how much pain they were causing. I left the group weighing much less, feeling my real body underneath my protective armor, loving it for the first time since I was two or three, wanting to dance naked again and feel the air on my wet skin.

4:00 P.M. Wellness with Ken. He says this group should be called the welling group because you never get wellness, you just move toward wellness. He can tell there's been a lot of heavy emoting going on in the groups today, and we talk about why we have to get in touch with our feelings here. When people are in trouble, pain, or fear, they unhook from their feelings to survive. But sooner or later their unhookedness makes it impossible for them to live. They're stuck in this unfeeling state, powerless, victims. Feeling again hurts, but it means that other feelings are possible, too, good feelings, pleasure. I think of how I've never really felt that—good, simple pleasure. Never had an orgasm. Suddenly I realize, of course not! How could I if long ago I unhooked myself from any kind of feeling, good or bad, to survive? Then I start thinking about what the future holds for me and it's not so painful after all. Being able to *feel* all sorts of things. Could that be what it means to be alive?

9 P.M. Called my husband and he wasn't home. Devastated to think he might be with another woman. I'm so vulnerable now. When the phone rang at ten and it was him, I felt like a schoolgirl. I asked him where he had been and he sounded hurt, as if he knew what was on my mind. "You know I've got an opportunity to make double overtime all this month," he said. I told him what Smitty recommended, about his coming down for family therapy. Right away he said, "I'll come." I was so glad I started blubbering again. "Elaine," he said, as if he were talking to a dense child. "I love you."

Day Eleven
CHOOSING A THERAPIST

If you have serious problems, it can be dangerous to think you can deal with them by yourself. Dissatisfaction with life, prolonged depression or anxiety, and a sense of helplessness are all indications of a need to go into therapy. I recommend group therapy for the following reasons: One, defenses are broken down quicker in group than in individual therapy. For instance, if you are blaming someone else for your problems, it's harder to argue with eight people than it is with an individual therapist, and there are a lot of individual therapists who will *never* challenge your point of view.

In one-on-one therapy a patient can easily get lost in mental abstractions. In a group the focus is on social interaction. Patients relate to each other's feelings, and the process of identification comes out of that. This process will not necessarily happen with individual therapists, particularly if they play a passive role and do not interact with their patients.

Another reason I recommend group therapy is the importance to recovery of a sense of belonging. Although you can get that sense of belonging from a 12-step fellowship, you can also hide out in one. You can get support you need from the fellowship, but no one will ever challenge you as a group will. There, confrontation is part of the growth process, with the therapist acting as a protector and moderator so no one gets scapegoated.

I also recommend group therapy because there is less of a chance for distortion to take place. In one-on-one, you may be taking on a therapist's issues and not even know it. For instance, a woman can end up with a male therapist who has a problem with his mother, who then gives a distorted perception of the patient's mother. Or, an anorexic might go to a therapist who didn't think she was underweight because of the therapist's own body-image distortions. Considering how many people have such distortions, I think you're a whole lot safer in a group. There, mirrored in the perceptions of six to eight other people, you have a better chance of learning to see yourself the way you really are.

Here are the qualities I believe are important to look for in choosing a therapist:

—*Truthfulness.* You need someone who will be direct and honest with you, so you don't have to guess what he or she means. Looking for someone who will tell you the truth is first on my list because it's so difficult for us to see ourselves the way we really are. The perceptions the therapist gives you will not necessarily mean it is "the truth," but at least you have a clear picture of how someone else perceives you, and a reality-based jumping-off place to work from. Some therapists are trained to give you nothing back, but to be a "mirror" on which you are to project your own feelings. I believe it's too easy to conceal ineptitude or indifference behind a mask of noninvolvement, and I prefer therapists who speak their mind rather than parrot back what you have just said, constantly asking you, "What do *you* think?" or (worse) saying nothing at all.

—*Direction.* Find a therapist who is willing to give

you suggestions. I believe people should ask for what they need and be specific about what they expect to happen. Then, if the therapist isn't willing to give you direction, cross him or her off your list and shop for one who will. (I give direction by encouraging my patients to take risks and change. Knowing how difficult that is, I understand when they don't, but the choice is still theirs to make when they're ready.)

—*Excitement*. I've had people tell me they have had therapists fall asleep in their sessions! Look in the eyes of your candidate and see if anybody is home. Look for a certain positive energy. If therapists don't exude a joy for living, I seriously wonder about their ability to help their patients develop one in themselves.

—*Nurturance*. You can teach professional techniques to therapists but you can't teach them to care. I am always disturbed when I meet members of my profession who really don't seem to care about people. Some of them have good insight, but I think it's more important for patients to be accepted and understood than given reasons why they behave in a certain way. I certainly wouldn't choose a therapist who didn't make me feel good about myself. In fact, I would avoid one who didn't at all costs! I value caring and being cared about higher than anything else, and I believe people intuitively know when someone is nurturing. Quite simply, it feels good to be around such a person. We all know inside when we meet a genuinely caring person. We can feel the energy. Trust your intuition if it's important to you to have a therapist of the nurturing kind.

—*Integrity*. If you discover a therapist doesn't give everyone in a group equal value, but gives preferential treatment based on social status, you have made a wrong choice. Everyone has the right to be treated with dignity, and I wouldn't trust a person who didn't practice that.

Group therapy is usually preceded by an intake interview and anywhere from one to five individual sessions before joining the group. At first, you should expect to feel uncomfortable. It's very anxiety producing to look at yourself honestly, so you can't use how you feel about the therapy as an indication of whether it's doing you any good. I tell people to commit themselves to ten sessions. If you just can't take it, at least go for five.

Bonding with a group can be a powerful experience. You may not ever be able to see yourself associating with the people in your group, or even liking them much, but the environment of shared vulnerability has the potential for creating a deeper kind of closeness than can happen in a friendship or even a relationship with a significant person. You are not in a group to cultivate friendships or please others, and that well-defined purpose allows you to focus on discovering who you really are and how to free that person imprisoned within you in order to live, **"happy, joyous, and free."**

Workbook for Day Eleven

ASSIGNMENT ONE

Draw up a list of the six qualities you need most in a therapist. If you have had previous experiences with therapists, evaluate them. Ask yourself, did the therapist make you feel like you could risk being vulnerable? Did you get direction? Did you lie to him or her? Most important, did you make progress? Then, describe in detail a nurturing person in your life whom you trust. Use the good feelings that person evoked in you as your guide when you seek a therapist.

ASSIGNMENT TWO

Find a buddy. Sit facing each other, knees touching, hands clasped. Look in your buddy's eyes and say, "I love you because . . ." until you run out of things to say. Then tell your buddy, "I fear . . ." until you run out of things to say. Your buddy then answers you, "I suggest . . ." Reverse roles. Be sure to maintain eye contact and loving thoughts.

You or your buddy may want to use this exercise whenever an urge to binge is strong, or when you are suffering from toxic thoughts. Hearing affirmations about yourself from someone you trust is a powerful and healing experience.

A Day in the Life
JEAN

Thursday, 7 A.M. I had a disturbing dream, but for the life of me I can't remember what it was about. I should keep my journal right by my bedside so I can write it down as soon as I wake up. This is the first morning I woke up on the first call. It wasn't easy, but I got up and I don't feel so groggy. My affirmation today: I am assertive, I am confident. I don't need people's approval. I approve of myself.

9 A.M. Gloria and I have a near altercation at breakfast. I try to sit down next to her and she snaps, "That's for Charlene," the anorexic she's so protective of. I want to punch her face in. She has such resentful eyes. Everyone's scared of her and she won't look at anyone. She's always stomping out of meetings, fiddling with things, coughing, and cracking her knuckles. She spills things, bumps things, and burned a big spot on purpose on the table with her cigarette. If we get blamed for that, I'm going to torture her. I'll get her in group. Nothing anyone says seems to affect her, but I'm not scared of her. She's going to hear from me because it's hard to be vulnerable around such an angry, resistant, self-indulgent, lazy bitch.

9 A.M. Step Study with Father Booth. I took good notes because I really felt he was talking to me: Addiction is repeating behavior in spite of the negative effects. Anything can become addictive. Workaholics feel powerless when not working. (I know that's true, because I see how frustrated Tony is here now that he's not allowed to make business calls. He paces the halls.) Watch out for other addictions developing once we have our food addictions arrested, such as going from a substance addiction to people addiction. Codependency is an addiction because addicts can't accept other people's need for space, and then codependency can lead right back to substance relapse. Sex addiction can be too much sex or none at all, just as anorexia is a food addiction—an addiction to not eating. Either way it's an obsession.

Father Booth says even religion can be addicting. (Wait till I tell my father that! I'd better wait until he's home from the hospital awhile.) He describes a religious addict as a victim of religious abuse—negative attitude, shame of body, isolation, low self-esteem, not allowed to question. There's a real danger of becoming narrow-minded—Jesus or else. Religious addicts can get addicted to evangelical TV personalities, gurus, cults. Many former atheists become religious nuts. He says, "Don't put us on a pedestal for our sakes as well as your own." God is not pleased the more you suffer. There comes a time when you have to say, "Hey, guys, time out for me." Don't give all to a church, work, this program, other people. It's what addicts do—all or nothing, everything in the extreme. I really felt like he was talking to me. I don't want to be an addict! But I know I am. It makes me so frustrated to face this about me!

11:30 A.M. I feel better after exercise. The instructor, Steve, is a staff member. He has a kind, easygoing, nonintrusive manner and is not too skinny or muscular, so he's not intimidating. He may be the most nonthreatening person I ever met. Anything you ask, he kind of smiles, looks off, and says, "Well," and then answers it in a clear, basic way. I'm glad I'm relaxed because underneath I'm nervous about group. I'm going to confront Gloria.

6:45 P.M. I didn't confront Gloria in group. We had words again at lunch. She said if I confronted her I should just fuck off or she'd explode. She started shaking all over and rattling her limbs at me. She loomed. I remained calm. I asked her what she was threatening me with and told her I wasn't scared of her. She abruptly changed the subject, saying she didn't want to talk about it. After lunch she kept throwing her garbage on my tray. I'm furious about that. I threw her napkin back at her, but she had already stormed off. I talked to Blanche privately and she said I should confront her in group and tell her what I need.

But I just didn't feel up to it. Instead, we discussed stealing in group. Everyone who will admit it has stolen because they thought they had nothing. It's a "fuck you" to those who do. Two people cried about the times they hit and verbally abused their children. They're both battered women and single parents themselves. I talk about how my mother is jealous of my sister and me, and how all three of us are manipulated by my father. I had to become the bad girl to stop playing the game. Blanche asked me, "What would happen if you stopped playing the bad girl *and* playing the game?" That made me think. I said, "You mean, I don't have to play the game?" Of course I know I don't, but I never even stopped to consider that.

I was ready to talk at the meeting tonight, but I didn't get called on. I was calm and I wanted to testify to my lifelong addictions, how I'm abstinent now, feeling the feelings, the pain, but having faith that I'm supposed to be doing this right now. I'm not frustrated that I didn't get to speak because listening was valuable. It just wasn't my day to get things off my chest, I guess.

I got this journal back from Blanche, and she wrote lots of comments. She wants me to explain my family role, and when I write nasty things about her, I'm supposed to tell her. She says I can be furious to her face and she won't leave me. I'm also supposed to tell people when they make me feel smothered, and talk about my sexual impulses. The more I'm quiet about them the more they run me. I'm to expose the game, the competition. What's the guilt about? What's behind my anger at Gloria? What are my feelings at night about sugar and alcohol cravings? What's the loneliness about? Do I worry? She reminds me of a teacher I had in the sixth grade. I wrote a journal for her, too, and she validated me the same way. No matter what I wrote, she said, "More." I thought I was really opening up in this journal, but I guess there's a lot I've been leaving out. I'm not used to this honesty. It's taken me all these years to get good at being devious. Being real is terrifying because I don't know how to be it, or who I'll be or what will happen.

Day Twelve

CODEPENDENCY AND ADDICTIVE RELATIONSHIPS

Codependency is a fairly new word, but it's a behavior trait as old as Adam and Eve. Dysfunctional families produce codependent behavior, which is defined in many ways: Codependence is focusing one's life on another person and calling it caring. It is doing things for others they can and should do for themselves. It is slavery by mutual agreement: two needy people don't want to focus on their own problems so they obsess on each other's. It's giving away your whole pie and leaving nothing for yourself.

My favorite definition of codependent people is: when they die, someone else's life flashes before their eyes!

"No man is an island." Everyone in this world is dependent on other people. Codependency is a matter of degree, and usually that degree is lopsided: one person gives 80 percent and the other 20. Here's a joke illustrating codependency: There was a mouse who asked an elephant if he could make love to her. She said, "Okay." While the mouse went at it, a coconut fell on the elephant's head. "Ouch," she said, and the mouse replied, "Oh! Did I hurt you?" That's a codependent talking.

No relationship is ever fifty-fifty all the time, but if the percentages are way off center, it's codependency—one is giving far too much and the other far too little. The person who cares too much is often staying in the relationship not because of the benefits derived from it but the fear of what would happen if faced with being alone. That fear far outweighs any pain suffered in the lopsided give-and-take of the codependent relationship.

The paradox is, in order for two people to be close, they have to be separate. The most comfortable relationship occurs when two people can live alone with each other. That's interdependency. If one needs the other too much, codependency results. If I must give up me to be loved by you, the price is too great. If I have never learned to love myself, I *can't* love you. That's the tragedy of most codependent relationships.

The subject of codependency comes up in the treatment of addiction because for many addicts it is the bottom-line obsession. I know many people who went into a 12-step program to stop drinking, only to become addicted to food. Then, when they went into recovery from that addiction, they turned to a relationship to obsess on. It's the addicts' dilemma to be constantly compelled to fill themselves up with an external. Relationships are the most difficult addiction of all; we don't expect food, alcohol, or other substances to love us back! We experience feelings related to love, but in relationships it's give, give, give.

Addicts have a tendency to codependent relationships. They may manage to function intellectually, and even be highly esteemed in their profession and in their community. Terrified they have no real identity of their own, they often bond with people who are emotional "takers" and are grateful for the chance to obsess on someone else rather than on their own seeming insignificance. They have a tendency to think the source of the stress is work or other external factors, but the source is always internal, and comes out of relationships.

No amount of relaxation techniques, meditation, assertiveness training, or affirmations will remove the stress caused by a codependent relationship. That doesn't mean we put off practicing them until recovery. We just have to know they are not going to take away stress. Only developing boundaries so that the flow of the relationship goes in as well as out will reduce stress to the degree of manageability.

Relationship addiction is really about someone else making you feel okay. It's needing another person to fill your cup. If you have low self-esteem and difficulty loving yourself, and if someone else is necessary to make you feel whole or alive, then you will undoubtedly suffer severe withdrawal symptoms if the loved one leaves, especially abruptly. It is then that the addiction can really be seen for what it is.

There are plenty of people caught up in relationship addictions, men and women alike. They go from one relationship to another, on emotional bender after emotional bender, to keep from having to face themselves and their terrifying inner emptiness. As someone I know pointed out, it's one thing to have a love affair with food or booze, but at least you don't expect it to call you on the phone.

I once knew an alcoholic who hid bottles all over his house, fearing that one day he would find himself without booze. That horrible day happened, on a Sunday when the liquor stores were closed. He walked for miles until, nearly crawling on his hands and knees in desperation, he found a bartender who sold him a bottle of vodka. Then, as soon as the bottle was in his possession, he was fine. He went home and didn't even take a drink. Having the alcohol in his house was more important than drinking it, and as soon as his relationship to the substance had been restored, he was all right again. That's what I see in many relationship addicts. It doesn't matter whether they're intimate with the object of their desires, they just need the body around to be okay. It's not who the person is that matters, it's just not being able to tolerate the state of being alone. If not being alone is your goal in life, you are undoubtedly a codependent, and you have most likely had a lot of difficulty establishing and sustaining relationships.

In gambling, anticipation of the game is more exciting than the actual act. It's a life-and-death situation, so the anticipation is more rewarding. The same thing happens with food: the anticipation of the act of eating it is more rewarding than the act itself. That also applies for relationships: the dreaming of what's going to happen is more rewarding than the actual relationship.

As long as other people are needed to form your identity, you will be living in an emotionally addictive state. As long as you are operating out of externals, where your identity comes from what you do or who you're with rather than who you are, you will never achieve the separateness that is necessary for two people to be truly intimate. Working on that identity is the last thing most codependents want, because they're so used to focusing on others. The thought of working on themselves fills them with despair, for it means a complete turnaround in their lifelong direction, and of relinquishing the idea of waiting for someone else to provide them with a sense of self. They hate having to face the realization that it won't ever happen.

When codependents decide to break free from their addiction to a relationship and seek their own identity, the people who depend on them to stay the same will do everything possible to change their minds. They will create emergencies, threaten to leave, and act out in all sorts of diverting ways. Because they will inevitably meet this opposition, codependents need help, and I believe the best kind available for codependency issues is group therapy. Although one-on-one therapy has its place, working out problems with a group helps unmask the incredible delusions that go along with relationship addictions. Hearing stories similar to your situation rather than your own voice session after session helps break through the denial process. It's hard to keep up the pretense when four or five people within a circle are telling your own story in your own words with different names for the same characters, and when you join them in the chorus of "me, too," it strengthens your resolve when you go home to bank the fires burning out of control as the people who had it so good when you were acting addictively desperately attempt to undermine the good you're doing for yourself.

Because their lives are so dependent on the feelings and reactions of others, codependents have a strong need for control and a basic lack of trust. They are great at trying to figure out why things happen, and they believe once they understand why, they'll be fixed. Often they will present the results of their ruminations to their therapist and feel judged when the therapist looks confused.

The hardest thing codependents ever have to do is stop figuring out what everybody else wants and start figuring out what they want. You're the only one who knows what it's going to take to make you happy. If you want it, go for it. If it's not right for you, God will stop you dead in your tracks—that's how you'll know what God's will is! But it will keep you in action instead of trying to make sense of everything *before* you take action.

Many new 12-step groups have formed around the subject of codependence. You may want to find a group that meets regularly to discuss your problems of codependency.

Workbook for Day Twelve

ASSIGNMENT ONE: PRAYER IS WHEN YOU SPEAK

"God grant me the serenity to accept the things I cannot change . . ."

List three situations in your life that you can't change and that you have difficulty accepting.

"The courage to change the things I can . . ."

List three situations in your life you are willing to change.

"And the wisdom to know the difference."

List three situations in your life that cause confusion because you are not sure whether you should accept them or try to change them.

Throughout the days to come, say the Serenity Prayer and ask for help with the specific situations you have listed. God will hear you the first time. It's your own attention you need to get, and repeating the requests will eventually reach that part of you so resistant to change. In the process of writing them down, you will begin to clarify for yourself exactly what it is you need to do.

A Day in the Life

TONY

Friday, 6:30 A.M. I woke up feeling lousy after a long phone conversation last night. My wife is going crazy dealing with my son. He's been threatened with expulsion from that high-class private school he goes to for skipping classes and generally fooling around. He seems to think my being in the hospital down here has given him license to go the limit. Between my son's acting up and my brother's prowling among the stockholders, I'd check out of here today if I weren't starting to feel better, a lot better. I know if I keep this up, it's going to do me some good.

Like I heard in one of the classes: Put anything before your recovery and you'll lose it. My wife really needs help, though. I want her to go to these Al-Anon meetings. Her father's a roaring alkie, her husband's a food addict, and she keeps saying, "I'm not the one with the problem. Why should I have to go to meetings?" She sounds depressed and harassed. So to make me feel better, what do I do? I call my sister, and she starts in on me about how her ex has just bought a red Ferrari. What's gotten into this guy? Do men go through change of life? I keep telling my sister she's got to build a life around herself, do some volunteer work, something, but she sounds just as hopeless as my wife. So then, I feel like I need a little support myself and I call Dad. He's in a funk about the business. Says he's tired of all this fighting among the relatives. Instead of making his life easier by retiring, he's opened Pandora's box. So all in all I feel just great today.

9 A.M. Step Study with Smitty. I'm starting to let go of my grip on surrender. Got to trust this program. I know something's working but don't know what it is. Food hasn't been on my mind since last Saturday when we went to Friendly's. I still can't believe I was sitting there surrounded by pictures of food and memories of a thousand pigouts drinking a Diet Coke. Just thinking about that makes me feel better.

1 P.M. Psychodrama was a two-bucket afternoon. I'm so wrung out I want to take a nap and skip the afternoon lecture. We number off and break up into small groups. I get Vickie, this counselor who doesn't miss a thing, I hear. They play this music, and we close our eyes and visualize our life as a movie, go back to moments when people hurt us, freeze the frame, and reach in and comfort ourselves. I froze the frame on a scene with my dad in his drinking days, coming home late one night after a real bender. Mom gets mad and he strikes her and I come roaring out, punch him with my fist. I'm only ten, and he throws me against the wall. The tears come and I'm a goner. As soon as this psychodrama stuff begins now I'm like Pavlov's dog, only instead of salivating it's tears. Then we're supposed to run the movie projector again, going through our lives, back in time, and then forward to the present, looking for people *we've* harmed, and before I know it I'm

in a freeze-frame with my son, age ten, hitting him with the back of my hand so hard he falls to the floor, my wife beating on me with her fists. I want to bolt out of there. Vickie starts going around the circle. Thank God she starts on the side opposite me, with this new guy who starts sobbing about the same thing, how he hit his kid with a belt. One after another I hear these stories of how people have hurt their kids, humiliated them, or hurt sisters, brothers, husbands, wives. The crying is different from when they let loose about having been abused themselves. This crying is like grieving, a terrible loss of something, maybe one's oh-so-great opinion of oneself. Then it's my turn and I'm no exception. I keep seeing that little boy I was and my son as the same person, like a perversion of the Golden Rule: "Do unto others as you have been done onto." God, this is so painful! How can I forgive myself for beating on my kid when I know how much I suffered having a dad who couldn't control his temper either?

Then Vickie tells us we can forgive ourselves. We can't do what we weren't taught. Victims victimize, and forgiving ourselves is not condoning the act, only letting go of it, to leave room for change. I was really scared of her, but I see now how effective she is, relentless but full of feeling. Then I see that in the process of forgiving myself I have to forgive others—my father, even my brother. He got the same beatings I did. He can't help he was the Golden Boy and I wasn't, that he was naturally gifted and I wasn't.

Afterward we form one large circle, twenty-four wasted, weeping, abused abusers, and they play that damn music that keeps the tears flowing like a faucet. We're supposed to keep our eyes closed and I feel someone's hands on my face, then whispering in my ear, "I forgive you, Tony." It's Vickie. "I forgive you. You're a good and loving person. You can heal." I bawl some more. Another person comes up, Blanche this time, then Smitty, who tells me to go around the group and forgive others. I open my eyes and seek out Elaine, who's just sobbing her heart out. I put my hands on her face and whisper in her ear, "I forgive you. You're a good person, Elaine, you can heal," and as I do so, some of the tension in my neck and shoulders lets go. I feel empty inside, then filled with a new, finer emotion. A powerful force is at work I don't understand, don't want to understand. I look around the room and find Jill, then Linda, then Jean, and Mike. We stand in the big circle again and I feel at one with them all.

Now I'm not tired anymore. I'm going to hear the lecture, not so much to hear it but to be with this group of all kinds of people I wouldn't normally get to know, let alone get close to, closer than I have ever felt to people in my life. Why is that? What's going on?

Day Thirteen

STEP STUDY: STEP TWO

"Came to believe that a Power greater than ourselves could restore us to sanity."

When mind and body are at war with each other, they can't work together. Sanity is when the mind, the body, and the spirit are all in harmony, a condition that is not possible as long as a person is in the throes of food addiction.

For years you may have been acknowledging a power greater than your own—your relationship with food. In this program you are asked to consider the possibility of the existence of another power greater than yourself that, unlike the demonic force of your addiction, does not exist to enslave you but to set you free. Step Two is about finding God in other people. It means acknowledging the power of the group is more powerful than we are, and that we can't do the job of restoring ourselves to sanity alone.

Personality change begins with Step Two, after taking the action of making a lifestyle change—that is, recognizing we need rituals for contact. In the process of that change, our values, attitudes, and beliefs will be held up to scrutiny and they will also change. The first to change will be what we value in life. The answer will now be obvious—other people. Those who had valued their isolation because it allowed them to indulge unchecked in their addictive behavior will no longer value it because minus the addiction, isolation is a painful state. There is no joy in it. Suddenly the value of other people, of a supportive group, will increase immeasurably. The attitude of "I can do it myself" will change to "I need other people."

Resisting help from others is resisting help from a higher power, for God works through other people. Faith in a higher power parallels how you trust people in your life. Control means you still don't have trust. As you begin to relinquish that control, you leave room for the power of the group to begin working in you.

Boundaries will also change. Energy will flow in both directions, between you and the fellowship. The power of love is one food addict helping another, and that power will help restore balance in other relationships—between family and friends, and in the workplace. Once the isolation is broken, the new intimacy you will have with the Real You will cause energy to flow in every direction, in every area of your life.

The restoration to sanity is a process. In it, first we come. Our feet bring us, and our unbelieving minds go along for the ride. Then we come to. We wake up. We start feeling. We came, we came to, and we came to believe, hardly an instantaneous event. It takes years for some, much less for others, depending on where they are when their feet first bring them to the process.

Coming to believe in a Power greater than ourselves is not necessarily a comforting thought. Any number of horror movies feature powers greater than ourselves. The miracle of the process is that this is a power greater than ourselves that *will restore us to sanity.* What a marvelous thought! The relief of being restored to sanity is greater than any gift a food addict could ask for.

The energy of intimacy, sharing of the Real Me, is the essence of the Second Step. In the sharing of the Real Me with others, a knowledge of God's energy within your own will protect you. You'll feel empowered, God protected, nurtured by intimacy. *You won't feel alone.*

The insanity addictive people feel has a lot to do with the abnormal stress patterns they experience. Normal stress looks like a wavy line—a steady flow of ups and downs. Addictive stress, on the other hand, looks like an erratic heart rate on a cardiologist's screen—constant ups and downs and finally collapse. At the point of collapse, people look around for a power greater than themselves to restore them to sanity. Some people turn to pills, and the pills usually have side effects. They make them anxious, so they have to take other pills to calm themselves. They in turn make them constipated, listless, dizzy, nauseous, paranoid, give them tremors, aches, vague feelings of foreboding. The pill takers are always worrying about running out of their prescriptions or not getting a new one filled in time, for they are unable to endure the thought of even a few hours without their pills.

There is only one side effect produced by the restoration of sanity in Step Two, and that is love. We arrive at it through hope and trusting our intuition. What we have been given, we must give back, and we are glad to do so. People are energy through which we can experience love and trust. Think of the infant. Without being able to say a word, it generates incredible energy and we are fascinated by its purity. We hold it and feel that energy transmitted to us. Similarly, without a word we encourage others in a state of insanity to seek help, for we bear witness that restoration is possible. We don't need to tell others that we have changed. By the clearness of our eyes and the peacefulness of our spirit, those who knew us when we were troubled will see for themselves that we have been restored to sanity. When we smile at them, we give them hope. We who were so hopeless a short time ago are now joyful, in harmony with ourselves and our surroundings. There is no pill in the universe that can produce this state of mind, only the power that promises to restore us to sanity.

Food addicts arrive at Step Two feeling disillusioned, angry, and betrayed. Have they gone through the pain and humiliation of admitting their powerlessness over food to be hit on the head with the need to believe in God? These days, it's easy to feel morally superior to the whole idea of religion. The ghastly religious wars of the Middle East make many people want to reject the idea of God altogether. In fact, the entire history of religion with its trail of blood and tears thousands of years in duration is enough to turn people away entirely.

No wonder so many people have problems with God.

Fortunately, God doesn't have problems with them. The God of the 12-step program has no ulterior motive, no hidden agenda, no temple that needs financing, no ring that needs to be kissed. You who have problems with God can decide the word stands for "good orderly direction," or that the power greater than yourselves is the power of the support group, or the power of this book if it's helping you feel better about yourself. The problems most people have with the idea of power is they have been taught to fear it, for it always implies power over—where the strong take advantage of the weak. The power of the 12-step program is never about power over. It's never something that needs to be feared. It empowers. It brings people from the state of powerlessness to being given power through others, by sharing the intimacy of who you really are. It's about becoming "happy, joyous, and free." It's about achieving a positive state of mind in which, wherever you are, whomever you're with, whatever you're doing, you will feel good about yourself because you know and love who you are, and because you will feel the presence of God in your life.

Sane people don't go on crusades. They just go about the business of living. Sane people don't have a yen to control your mind. They've learned they don't want to control anything, not even their own minds. They've learned to give up the entire idea of control and to wait in that naked and vulnerable state for a power greater than themselves that will give them something much better than they could ever have created on their own, something they most likely have never even experienced, or felt only in small moments of bliss.

The precious gift of awareness is waiting for those who come to believe. There is no price to pay, no pledge of allegiance, no vows, no dues or initiation fees, no contracts to sign. All that is required is belief, and somehow that comes. Sometimes it seems to come of its own accord. The power we seek does not always manifest itself in a shaft of light, although that happens. I have heard too many sane, normal, ordinary people tell about that experience to doubt it. The power manifests itself when we pray not for what we want but merely for the power to carry out God's will for us, having the faith of a mustard seed.

Belief is a matter of "reliance, not defiance." It does not tell God what to do and then get angry when it doesn't happen. That you have to give up your list of demands—what your own will thinks you want—may seem the most bitter pill of all to swallow, but I can assure you God's will for you is like a surprise gift containing something you didn't even know you wanted but badly needed and never thought to ask for, and never dreamed could be yours. The room for surprise once you step out of God's way is one of the most intriguing aspects of this program. The power that comes when you ask for knowledge of God's will is another. Following it is so easy, like having the wind at your back instead of fighting it every inch of the way. There is little more I can say until you experience for yourself that there is a healing power greater than your own, except my constant reassurance that help is on the way, if you will just keep going in the direction you're in. The disease of addiction is a detour from the person we were meant to be. Recovery is a discovery process of who that wonderful person really is through a personal revelation of God's will for you.

The experience of slogging on without reason to believe is called faith, and it is a state of grace. In that protective state, faith will carry you until your first tangible results that this program works. How will you know when it starts working? You will *feel* it, and that feeling will be all the proof you will need to continue.

Workbook for Day Thirteen

ASSIGNMENT ONE

Draw a picture of the God of your childhood. Describe your relationship with that God. Draw a picture of a higher power that you would like to believe in. Do you believe there is or might be a power greater than yourself? If not, do you wish you could believe there was a power greater than yourself? If you are still filled with doubt and despair, are you willing to continue reading this book in spite of your objections to the "God stuff"? Be honest. The only one this answer is important to is you. God will wait.

A Day in the Life
ELAINE

Saturday. When I got up I said "Good morning" to Gloria and she said, "How do you know?" Later on she barked at me, "What time is it?" And I said, "Now." She laughed like a little kid.

Noon. By the duck pond. I have always seen myself as the Big Giver. Thursday in group I brought up how mean Jean treats me, that every time I reach out to her she draws back and says things like, "You're in my space," and instead of agreeing with me about Jean, I found out most people don't relate to me as a giver at all but go to others when they need some comfort, and I'm devastated by that. They see me as a victim—someone needy—a taker, not a giver! Tim said I smile too much. Kathryn said I can just be myself (implying "whoever that is . . ."). Even Mary intimated she thinks I try too hard to be liked. The only one who made me feel good was Tony. He tried to soothe things over, said he thought I was a great person just the way I was. Suddenly I am stripped of my identity. I don't think they or anyone likes me, and of course that's so terribly important, to be liked by one and all! If I can sit with this feeling long enough, I'm hoping that need can lose some of its importance. Can't I be like a duck in this pond floating along enjoying the sunshine and the coolness of the water? Is it so important to win this popularity contest? The thing is, I know deep down that I don't give a damn about others, not really, and just give the appearance of it. I'm too locked up in my shell of self-protection tending to my image of Helpful Hanna to give more than a superficial shit what's going on with the rest of the world.

When I told Smitty my husband said he was coming for group therapy, he asked me, "How about your children?" I lied and didn't tell him I forgot to bring it up. Why did I forget? Don't I want them to come? Or am I afraid they won't want to come, that I don't matter? I mean, what if I'm not worth it? I feel so horrible. Three days ago when I did that powerful work in group, remembering that incident of being hit with the broom, I felt awful and then I felt so peaceful, like I was really getting better. Now I feel worse than ever. I really can't take this place.

Jill just came in and asked me if I want to go to the mall on our Saturday pass. When people were making arrangements at breakfast, I didn't say anything because I was afraid no one would want to spend their Saturday afternoon with phony me. Now I feel a little bit better. So foolish that a grown woman with children should feel like an adolescent when I walk into the lunchroom, worrying about where I should sit, not wanting to offend anyone! It's like I never learned how to act sociably. I feel about thirteen today.

10 P.M. Talked to Danny. Asked him if he would like to come for family therapy with his dad next weekend. He said he'd talk to him about it and let me know. Kathleen is with her boyfriend. Ever since psychodrama, when I realized I had been as distant to my kids as my mother had been to me, there but not really present, I feel so bad about myself. I don't know who I am.

Day Fourteen

WHAT'S EATING YOU CAN ALSO MAKE YOU SICK!

The link between mental attitude and physical illness is finally being taken seriously by the medical establishment, and in the past decade a whole new field of study called psychoneuroimmunology, a combination of the fields of psychology and immunology, has emerged. During the 1980s, research conducted by the National Institute of Mental Health, New York's Mt. Sinai Hospital, and other major institutions has documented surprising new evidence that employment of the techniques used in this book to change a person's self-defeating state of mind—stress-reducing relaxation therapies, moderate physical exercise, visualization, cognitive restructuring, meditation, positive affirmations, and confronting traumatic memories—actually enhances the body's immune system. The new studies confirm what many already believed—that people who think sick are more likely to be sick.

and that people who think well are more likely to be well.

The concept that emotions affect physical health has been around in medical circles for a long time. In the second century A.D., a Greek physician noted that unhappy women were more prone to develop cancer than happy women, and a belief that psychic imbalance (the four humors) caused disease was central to the practice of medicine in Europe until the rise of modern science in the seventeenth century. After that, however, the relationship between emotions and physical health was given as much credence among medical practitioners as witch doctors and faith healers. It is only in the last decade that we have seen a surprising turnaround in their thinking. Hundreds of studies have now been done that show that a person's state of mind affects the immune system.

These days, protecting your immune system is as important as getting a polio vaccination was in the 1950s, for our bodies' natural line of defense is under attack from many sources—AIDS and other viruses that attack the immune system such as Epstein-Barr, herpes, and Chronic Fatigue Syndrome, plus cancer, environmental contaminants, and high levels of stress.

In order to understand how we can help our immune system, we need to take a look at how that system works. It is a marvel of complexity, much of it still a mystery. A healthy immune system operates much like a well-disciplined army. The first line of defense is at the skin level. A wound or lesion will be surrounded by swarms of phagocytes, white blood cells that eat the transgressing bacterial cells until the phagocytes die in the process, forming the yellow-white substance commonly known as pus around the wound.

The secondary line of defense are the lymphocytes, such as B-, T-, and natural killer cells. They roam the bloodstream searching for antigens, foreign substances such as bacteria, viruses, or toxins. The lymphocytes then release antibodies, which destroy the invader.

Endorphins are the link between the immune system and the brain. They are neurotransmitters such as serotonin, acetylcholine, and norepinephrine, compounds that act like messengers shuttling electrical impulses between the nerve cells in the brain, triggering a highly complex response that begins in the hypothalamus and ends in the cells of the immune system. Recent discoveries have found that these neurotransmitters also play a role in controlling the autonomic nervous system, the part that operates automatically to regulate all the involuntary activity of the body. This connection between the autonomic nervous system and the immune system has caused the scientific community to completely rethink its position on how the body protects itself. The new research also shows that these messages can be communicated in both directions. Some of the neurotransmitters, such as the "feel good" opiate betaendorphin, originate in the immune system itself. In fact, these mood-altering transmitters have recently been found in all parts of the body, not just the brain! The idea of a feedback loop, that the central nervous system can influence the immune system, which can then influence the central nervous system, is creating much interest and excitement among researchers, and it further illustrates the biochemical linkages between body and mind.

Since the pioneering work of Dr. Hans Selye in the 1950s, hundreds of studies have been conducted that confirm his original research on the effects of emotional stress on the immune system, that neurotransmitters produced in the brain travel through the blood to alter the activity of the immune system on the cellular level. Not all stress is damaging. In fact, mild forms of stress can actually enhance the immune system, but unhealthy levels, particularly acute stress, can weaken it. Fear and rage, or inappropriate triggering of the fight-or-flight syndrome (which provided our ancestors with the adrenaline needed to escape from wild beasts but is of little help when confronting an angry spouse or boss), are the kinds of stress that do people harm. Unhealthy stress decreases the body's protein and fat synthesis and glucose use, diminishing the amount of insulin it produces. It also creates a biochemical domino effect that begins in the brain with an increase in the production of the hormone corticosterone, which in turn decreases the number of

T-cells, B-cells, and natural killer cells, which patrol the immune system, destroying newly formed cancer cells and other invaders.

A major study conducted at New York's Mt. Sinai Hospital documented the impairment of the immune system in men whose wives had recently died. Their bereavement impaired the ability of their lymphocytes to destroy intruders. A study done there in 1984 on people hospitalized for depression documented a decline in the number of lymphocytes in their bloodstream.

Studies have also been done on the effects of alcohol on the immune system, and they convincingly show that it inhibits the response of the immune system's defense mechanisms, predisposing the heavy drinker to infection.

So far, the effects of positive mental states on the immune system have not been as well documented as the effects of negative mental states. In 1976, Norman Cousins's book describing how he overcame ankylosine spondylitis, a chronic, progressive disease of the spine, with vitamin C and laughter was interesting but anecdotal as far as the medical community was concerned. Bernie Siegel's books on the subject helped millions. By the 1980s, hundreds of carefully controlled studies have found conclusive evidence that there is a strong link between mental attitude and physical health.

Stress-reduction techniques have been found to lower blood pressure, the rate of respiration, and the triggering of the "fight-or-flight" response in the autonomic system, which other studies have found impairs the functioning of the immune system. Another study found that when subjects were hypnotized and given a suggestion that their white blood cells were like sharks devouring tiny fishlike antigens, the activity of their lymphocytes actually increased. Serotonin levels have been found to increase with the use of brain synchronizers, gadgets with flashing lights that are worn like sunglasses during meditation. Raising endorphin levels is bound to make anyone feel better, particularly the genetically addicted, whose endorphin levels are lower than average.

A study on people at risk for AIDS found that a combination of exercise, relaxation therapy, and stress-management techniques increased the number of their T-4 cells, which fight infection and viruses and decrease once the AIDS virus begins to progress. Physical exercise has long been believed to improve a person's resistance to infection, but many recent studies show that extreme forms of exercise are actually an immunosuppressant. Vitamins, on the other hand, enhance the function of the immune system. In one study, supplements of vitamin E and C were given to adults joining an exercise program. Others were given placebos. At the end of six months, there was a significant increase in the number of T lymphocytes in the immune systems of people given the vitamin supplements.

Most interesting to me are the recent findings that have led researchers to postulate that people who are out of touch with their emotions, or unaware of them, or who are unable to express them, particularly the negative ones, are more susceptible to a suppression of the defense capabilities of their immune systems. One study involved volunteers writing down their most traumatic experiences and describing their feelings about them. Many of the subjects had never discussed these experiences of family violence, sexual abuse, suicide attempts, and other upsetting events with anyone. For four days in succession, writing for twenty minutes each day, the study showed a surprising increase in their levels of T-cells. Because food addicts are so good at stuffing down their feelings, they are particularly susceptible to suppression of their immune system's capabilities. Knowing they are actually improving their body's defenses while they are healing emotionally and growing spiritually is one more strong motivation for change.

I am excited about the research that is now going on in the connection between mental state and the immune system, for it takes the whole concept of behavioral medicine out of the realm of superstition and fits it squarely into that of Western medicine. Now, instead of wasting energy on disputing the connection, researchers can concentrate their energies on which behavioral therapies produce the greatest benefit, and on ways to use psychoneuroimmunology in the prevention of disease. Although pharmacologists have yet to produce a synthetic endorphin, we can learn to increase the manufacture of it in our brains by applying the techniques spelled out in this book. They are now all scientifically proven to increase the ability of our immune systems to keep us healthy.

Workbook for Day Fourteen

ASSIGNMENT ONE

Although it is not possible to monitor the results, it is possible to replicate the aforementioned study on confronting emotional trauma and its benefits on the immune system. For the next four days, spend twenty minutes each day writing about the most traumatic event in your life. If you are in therapy, show the results to your therapist. If you are not in therapy, share it with someone you are close to and trust.

A Day in the Life

JEAN

Sunday. My affirmation for today: to acknowledge the great investment I have made in this program, and how terrific I am that I am trying to change. My stay here is half over. I can't believe the time has gone so fast, but I feel I haven't really gotten down to business. I get distracted too easily. My dreams are so disturbing, but by the time I wake up they're gone. I'm left only with this awful panicky feeling. Other people around me are really getting down to business, like Debbie. She's working hard in Vickie's group about her problems with her husband. Yesterday Smitty told her, "Don't smile, Debbie. It's addictive. It gets to feeling good and it might screw up your depression." That was the first time she had smiled in about a week. Elaine isn't smiling anymore either. I think she's getting down to business, too. When will I?

5:30 P.M. I learned something. Tim told me he was angry that I moved his clothes from the washer, and we're not supposed to do that. I let him tell me, said I was sorry, but didn't feel *bad*. I'm not thinking, "Oh, no, now he doesn't like me so I have to be uncomfortable around him." I know he was just practicing his assertiveness by expressing his feelings directly. I'm glad he told me instead of someone else, but I had my own reasons for moving his clothes.

5:40 P.M. Tim lied. That's not a rule. Do I call him on it? It's not a big deal, but he should know I don't like people being dishonest. He should also be aware of his own wash cycle.

In our afternoon meeting we sang Happy Birthday to Mary and shouted in unison, "Congratulations! You're a celebration of life," and she burst into tears. We said the congratulations to Gloria who was sitting down (she refused to stand up), and she ran out of the room. I wonder what her problem is. She never has a thing to say in group.

7 P.M. I feel relaxed. I called Tim on the laundry flap and he just shrugged his shoulders and said, "Sorry." Things are fun socially. We were laughing on the bus and playing like kids. Tim was massaging Debbie's shoulder and I said, "I miss men's shoulders. I'm so horny." Tim invited me into the massage train. It felt great to be touched. We have all these sexual jokes and a place for the energy to go. Laura, one of the older women, glares at us. I guess she thought we were having too much fun.

Debbie came in just to talk. She had tears in her voice so I encouraged her to stay. She's having the same problems I am, feeling guilty about wanting to be with certain people more than others. One of the patients here actually confronted her, telling her she felt she didn't get enough attention from her. Poor Debbie. That comment ruined her whole day. It's so controlling—"Like me, now." We decided it's not her problem. I'm going to say something to these aggressive codependents next time, such as, "You're in my space" or something. Debbie and I decide it's not realistic to like everyone. We both feel better. I think we did it without gossiping, tried anyway, but as soon as I say someone's name or hear it said when they're not in the room, it feels like gossip. It's hard to be honest.

9 P.M. I called my parents. My father is home. His voice sounds weak. Mother is a little too cheerful. She

says she hopes I'm finding out what's wrong with me. I hang up wondering why I ever call them. I always end up feeling lousy when I do. So then I call my sister. She sounds worried. I ask her what's wrong and she actually tells me—says Patti, her eight-year-old, is having trouble at school. She keeps falling asleep in class. They've taken her to the doctor and he can't find anything wrong with her. "She won't eat," my sister says, and starts crying. "Did you do that when you were little? I don't remember."

I tell her no, trying not to get sarcastic, and bite my tongue to keep from saying she shouldn't worry. I don't have a contagious disease. I suggest that she not make a big deal out of whether she eats or not.

When I hang up, I actually feel close to my sister. I don't think she's ever been honest with me before. She always puts up such a front that everything is all right. We were bred to compete, and you never reveal a weakness to your competitor. It tells me that we're starting to free ourselves from the need to play the family game.

3 A.M. I wake up screaming. Jill is right by my side. "What's the matter?" she says. "Did you have a bad dream?" A nurse comes running in. They sit on either side of me on my bed and encourage me to remember, but I don't need encouragement. The dream is too vivid for that. Finally I get it out. I'm lost. Everything so dark and foreboding, houses looming, or maybe doorways, and then there's a man. He's standing over me. I don't know who he is. Can't see his face. But I can see his penis, huge and erect, dangling between his legs, moving toward my face.

"I think you've had a flashback," the nurse tells me. "Events you've suppressed are starting to come out in dreams. Don't be afraid. Now you're really getting somewhere."

I don't want to go back to sleep because I'm afraid I'll dream it again, or another one. I know there's more. The dream has a strong feeling of being a preview, just an introduction to a horror show. I take my notebook and sit at the little table by the nurses' station and start writing my autobiography, going back to my earliest memory, and find out I don't have any, nothing at all, until about the age of ten. Blanche will have a lot to say about that. I think of her and feel warm. She will help me. I thank God for her. I have her voice inside me right now, assuring me that everything is going to be all right.

6

Week Three

Letting Go

Two weeks of healthy eating and abstinence from mood-altering substances are beginning to have a positive effect on your state of mind. Your mood is more even and tranquil; your highs are less high, your lows less low. You are beginning to experience real emotions, and wondering what to do about them. Week Three concentrates on expressing those emotions and then letting them go.

Two weeks of moderate daily exercise are also beginning to make you feel better about yourself. Your muscle tone is improving, more oxygen is reaching your cells, flushing out toxins and clarifying your thinking. The muscles in your legs are becoming more defined and you have fewer aches and pains.

Two weeks of meditation and positive affirmations are also beginning to have a good effect, giving you enough security to examine your behavior and identify what defenses you have been using to protect yourself, and the courage to discard them.

Every now and then the real you comes out of prison and has a look around. More and more that person will dare to step forth, increasingly confident that he or she won't be abused or ignored. You know when your true self is present because you feel blissfully authentic, totally in the moment, and that moment is serene even when the activities around you are in chaos. It is the state you are striving to be in all the time, so you can be truly alive. You don't have to prove anything. Facts have little to do with the state you seek. Spirituality comes out of feeling, not logic. It moves from guesswork, intuition, feelings.

Day Fifteen
CHILDHOOD SEXUAL ABUSE

I define sexual abuse as any behavior that causes people to feel fear, shame, and a sense that something is wrong with them. Its prevalence among children is society's "dirty little secret." Nationwide, studies indicate around 16–17 percent of the population have been sexually abused as children. Studies conducted on people with eating disorders reveal a much higher percentage than in the general population. In a survey of five hundred people who have gone through Janet Greeson's "A Place For Us," 27 percent said they were incest survivors. A study by Father Leo Booth documents the same percentage among nuns. In the broader category of sexual abuse (including acts committed by people outside the family) the statistics are truly shocking. In one survey of patients with eating disorders, 64 percent said they had undergone coercive sexual events as children. Seventy-five percent was the statistic given on the television special on the subject of eating disorders called *Kate's Secret* starring

Meredith Baxter Birney, and I have read other studies that claim a figure among the addict population as high as 80 percent.

There is a logical reason for the high incidence of sexual abuse among people with eating disorders. Food is usually the only mood-altering substance available to children, and they turn to it for solace to numb their feelings of rage and shame. Many develop a lifelong emotionally charged relationship with food that eventually leads to an eating disorder. Among people with eating disorders, the incidence of sexual abuse is the highest among bulimics. It is, after all, a disease of secrecy.

One of the most damaging aspects of childhood abuse is this element of secrecy. Bruno Bettelheim made the observation that when the pattern of abuse among children is societal—the unfortunate "norm"—they do not take on the guilt of their oppressors. Children abused out in the open, particularly when it is a fate they see shared by others, suffer far less psychological damage than children who were abused in private. Secrecy distorts reality and makes the child take on the blame and the shame the oppressor should be feeling. These feelings are then turned inward on themselves because they have nowhere else to go, and fear of discovery keeps the feelings buried, because as children they were frequently threatened into remaining silent or convinced what happened was their fault.

In order to escape from an intolerable situation, the sexually abused develop disassociating mechanisms, taking leave of their bodies to live in their heads. Some take leave of reality itself and develop multiple personalities. Others simply learn to "go away," to leave their bodies mentally and emotionally. The ultimate abandonment is the forced exile from the self, and it is the tragic legacy of childhood sexual abuse.

Although all forms of sexual abuse are abhorrent, incest is the most damaging because it occurs within the family circle where children are supposed to be safe from harm. In the case of incest by a parent, the event may be so traumatic it is completely repressed, or children may create a self-protective myth out of the incident that *they* are responsible for the behavior of the parent. Because they cannot survive knowing the parent they depend on for nurturance is also abusing them, they take on the parent's guilt and minimize what happened, or repress it entirely, often disconnecting from their bodies in the process. Many never get reconnected. One of my patients with a long history of deep depression had been to six treatment centers before coming to Janet Greeson's "A Place For Us." At none of them had the issue of incest even been addressed, let alone pursued. When she felt safe enough at the center, she let herself remember, and her lifelong depression has since lifted. She came back from exile and is living in her body again, able to feel both pleasant and hurtful emotions. Getting reconnected doesn't mean the end of feeling bad, just the beginning of feeling anything.

It is amazing to me how many of my sexually abused patients come from very religious homes. The incidence of incest is unusually high among the highly religious, as if the unnatural damming up of the sexual urge common among them causes desperate people to seek other outlets. All too often the outlet of least resistance is a child. Sexually abused children must learn to live somehow with contradictory moral messages. They are often taught that sex is bad, and that they should watch out for strangers. Yet a relative does the bad thing to them, often the same person who said it was wrong. In an attempt to make sense of the hypocrisy, children create explanations for themselves in which reality becomes badly fractured.

Traditionally, rape victims were blamed for their victimization, and the same holds true for children who are sexually molested. They must have "asked for it," especially if they were desperate for affection and attention. I know one five-year-old girl who begged to go to confession to relieve herself of her guilt after being sexually abused by an older brother. Survivors of sexual abuse must be told again and again that they are not responsible for what was done to them.

When sexually abused children grow up, they continue to live in a state of altered reality, using food or drugs to dull the troublesome feelings they can't control or comprehend and that won't go away. If you were sexually abused as a child and have not dealt with the issue, you need help. If you are wondering whether you have repressed memories of sexual abuse, believe me, no one makes up such an unhappy past for him- or herself. The seeds can be planted in someone's mind, but they will not germinate if the event didn't take place. If you have a secret you're keeping from yourself, your autonomic nervous system will respond to the memory prodding and begin to work on bringing up all the repressed emotions that must be dealt with.

You cannot deal with this issue alone. There is a profile of a survivor of childhood sexual abuse in today's workbook section. If your identification with it is high, I strongly recommend you go into therapy. If you can't, there are sexual abuse hotlines and 12-step Incest Survivor and Adult Children of Alcoholics groups all over the country. Contact one in your area.

Workbook for Day Fifteen

ASSIGNMENT ONE

The past only matters in how it's affecting you today. Today you are going to write a story that will help you clarify that connection. It is a short story, consisting of three paragraphs. The first paragraph begins "Once upon a time," and it tells how someone, yourself or a fictional character, or even an animal, protected him- or herself in the past. The second paragraph begins "When he/she grew up" and tells how that person continued the behavior learned in the past. The third paragraph begins "The story changed when" and tells how that person learned different patterns of behavior to cope with life. It will reveal how you would feel about yourself with a new style of interacting compared to the old style that didn't work, and it will begin motivating you to put that new style into practice.

ASSIGNMENT TWO: PROFILE OF A SURVIVOR OF CHILDHOOD SEXUAL ABUSE

Check off the characteristics that are true for you:

1. ____ You have no memory of childhood, or only brief flashes, such as being held on someone's lap.
2. ____ You feel guilty a lot for no reason.
3. ____ You have a history of inability to sustain a love relationship.
4. ____ You frequently indulge in short pursuit-and-revenge love affairs, earning a reputation for being a Jezebel or a "lady killer."
5. ____ You consistently find the excitement of a triangular love affair (for instance, involvement with someone who is married) more exciting than involvement with someone who is available.
6. ____ You experience flashbacks in a waking state: brief, vivid, and disturbing images of a sexual nature that provoke strong anxiety.
7. ____ You have recurring dreams of a sexual nature, often involving body parts or unidentified people, that provoke strong anxiety.
8. ____ You have difficulty establishing boundaries, either letting everyone in or keeping everyone out.
9. ____ You practice all-or-nothing extremes in sexual behavior such as celibacy or promiscuity.
10. ____ You are often strongly drawn to people who abuse you.
11. ____ You are obsessed with love relationships and only feel alive when seeking or receiving affection.
12. ____ You feel disconnected from your body, as if it were numb from the neck down.
13. ____ In order to achieve orgasm, you often fantasize scenes of bondage where you are coerced into the sexual act.
14. ____ You have an excessive need to please.
15. ____ You practice self-mutilation, scratching or cutting yourself until you bleed, either consciously or in your sleep.
16. ____ You have a problem with moral ambivalence and often seek the opinion of others about a moral issue because you don't trust your own.
17. ____ You are overly protective of others.
18. ____ You are manipulative rather than assertive in dealing with others.

19. ____ You fear the consequences of change.
20. ____ You are uncomfortable when good things happen to you and become anxious if good feelings are prolonged.
21. ____ When you were young, you felt older than your peers and never really felt like a child.
22. ____ You have magical expectations of other people and the world.
23. ____ You have abnormally high expectations of yourself that you can't possibly meet.
24. ____ You have a pattern of failure in meeting and satisfying your own needs.
25. ____ You expect people to read your mind. (Please guess my awful secret.)
26. ____ As a child you felt special and believed you were the favorite.
27. ____ You have a tendency to "space out."
28. ____ You are secretive and have trouble trusting others.
29. ____ You generally feel inauthentic, or as if you wear a mask.
30. ____ You have a great desire to dance but are inhibited and can't let go.
31. ____ You have a strong identification with the oppressed and are active in human rights or animal rights causes.

If you checked more than twenty of the characteristics, you need to consider finding someone to help you. Not thinking you are worthy of giving yourself something you really need is part of the profile. (See Day Eleven, Choosing a Therapist.)

ASSIGNMENT THREE: MIRROR AFFIRMATION

This is a powerful affirmation, and it will assist you in bringing up repressed memories. If you fit the above profile of a survivor of childhood sexual abuse, do not use it unless you are getting some kind of therapeutic help.

Look directly into your eyes and repeat this affirmation three times, in the morning and again at night before you go to bed:

[Call yourself by name], you are wonderful and
I love you.
This is one of the best days of your life.
Everything is working for your greatest good.
Whatever you need to know is revealed to you.
Whatever you need will come to you.
All is well.

A Day in the Life

TONY

Monday, 7 A.M. Got weighed today. I've lost another six pounds. Grand total: nineteen! Wow, I feel so great. And the best part is, I haven't felt deprived. I know it won't be as easy on the outside because I'll have to make choices, but I really feel good about myself.

10 A.M. Step Study. I love Smitty. He says, "God don't make junk."

1 P.M. I read my letter to my brother in group today and nothing happened. It might as well have been a grocery list. Instead of getting any feelings out I sort of imploded. Now I feel physically sick and disappointed. It's like I brought all this garbage to the dump and instead of dumping it, I put it in my car and brought it back home. Now it stinks to high heaven. I know these old pent-up feelings are poisoning me. I can feel it! Smitty said I need to ask my brother to come down for family therapy. I hate to do that, but I know I've got to. Damn it! Why do men have such a hard time of it. The women in the group just bawl at a moment's notice. The only man I've seen here really let loose is my roommate, Sam, and he's wild and out of control anyway. I don't know what I think I'll lose if I got any feelings out. My dignity? Some dignity walking around like Porky Pig.

3 P.M. Wellness lecture with Ken. He was talking about magical thinking, and it brought back my childhood in a big way, like thinking, if I can hold my breath all the way to the telephone pole, I can get an A on my social studies test. He says when kids live in an untrustworthy environment they go inside and reinvent it so it feels like we have some control over it. But I know I still do it, and

Ken just made that connection for me. When my wife was in the hospital, I was playing those crazy "If I do this, then that will happen" games with myself. Ken tells us people come into treatment centers because they think there's something terribly wrong with them. What's wrong is they're honest and they can't lie as well as everyone else. He says, "I like coming here because it's one of the few places in my life that I find honest people. I don't feel crazy in here. I feel crazy out there."

8 P.M. Called my brother. I can't believe he said he's coming down, just like that. He says there's a lot of things he's always wanted to say to me, too. When he said that, I got a sick feeling inside. Family group therapy is a forum of sorts, and lots of people will be making comments on how we interact, people I trust. What if they take his side? Well, whatever. I'm in for it now.

Day Sixteen

HELPING YOUR INNER CHILD

When we were children we were playful and spontaneous. What happened? Some of us have forgotten how to play because of messages we learned about how we "should" or "ought" to be. But the child we were is still alive within us and we can teach it new messages. In gratitude, that child will come out and teach the adult in us how to be playful, creative, and spontaneous. But first that child of yours has to learn to trust you. He has been abused or neglected by you. How many times have you scolded yourself out loud? Your inner child takes that to heart and feels wounded. She may be wondering if anyone will ever come and rescue her. If you want to rescue your inner child, you need to remember that you have not done much over the years to inspire trust.

We speak to that inner child through visualization, as children respond more readily to pictures than words. For that reason, this explanation is short today, like a child's attention span, so you can go right to work on communicating with your child in pictures.

Workbook for Day Sixteen
THE INNER CHILD

ASSIGNMENT ONE: VISUALIZATION

Choose a time when you can be alone and uninterrupted. Find a photograph of yourself as a child, preferably one that is full face, in which you can see your eyes. If you have a record or tape of environmental music of ocean sounds, play it softly in the background, or play some beautiful and soothing music of your choice.

Sit comfortably with the photograph on your lap and begin meditating the way you have been practicing. When your mind is quieted, pick up the photograph of yourself and focus on that small face. Look directly into the eyes of that little child. Then close your eyes and see the face in your mind. See what your inner child is wearing. Notice the setting: Is your child hiding? You may have to coax it to come forward. Is it sitting or standing? What kind of expression is on its face? As you see that child, allow yourself to have compassion in your mind's eye, and then step into the scene and put your arms around your child. Let it know you're there and that it's important to you. Now pick your child up and speak soothingly. Ask your child, "What did you need to hear but never did?" When you hear the answer, tell your child that now. Let your child talk to you freely about its pain, and when it has told you everything it needs to tell you, ask what it needs.

When you hear the answer, give your child what it needs at once, either emotionally or symbolically. Then take your child's hand and go for a walk by the ocean. Enjoy the feel of the sand beneath your feet and the breeze on your cheeks. Listen to your child the way you wanted to be listened to when you were little. Let your child know how much you love it and that you will always be there.

ASSIGNMENT TWO: A LETTER FROM YOUR INNER CHILD

Using your nondominant hand, write a letter from your inner child to your adult self, expressing whatever feelings come to mind. With the dominant hand, write as an adult to your child, acknowledging the child's pain. Begin to nurture and comfort it. You and your child may begin a dialogue, or you may be more comfortable with letters.

The nondominant hand creates a pipeline to the inner child, circumventing the mind-set of the adult. You may want to use it whenever you feel out of touch with your child, or when you are feeling good about yourself and want to send it an extra dose of comfort and love.

A Day in the Life
JEAN

Tuesday, 9 A.M. Last night I had a recurring dream: I'm in the house on Orchard Street. The door opens to the pantry. I see jars of canned peaches and tomatoes. That much I've had over and over for years. This morning I have the rest: a man looming over me, then body parts. Horrible. Then a face, my uncle's face, his twisted smile. I woke up when it was still dark and went into the bathroom and threw up, dry heaves. There wasn't anything in my stomach. I feel so sick. My whole body is throbbing, and my stomach aches, like I've had food poisoning.

9:30 A.M. I was shaking so bad I couldn't sit in the step study class. Went looking for Blanche and found her in her office. She held me and told me I wasn't going to die, that these were the feelings I would have had when I was abused but couldn't express because I was afraid. Now my body knows I'm safe and is taking charge. I just have to be willing to go with my feelings and to trust them.

1 P.M. I tell group about my dream, and the man who now has the face of my uncle. Gloria, that bitch, makes a gesture like she's trying to make herself throw up by jamming a finger down her throat. I start screaming at her. I want to tear her apart! Blanche tries to get Gloria to explain what her gesture means, and finally she says, real nonchalant, "So, big deal. My dad sticks it to me every chance he gets." Well, I was so mad that Gloria took the focus off my problem to finally reveal just what it is that

makes her so crazy that I didn't care a bit about her tragedy! Then Gloria clammed up again and wouldn't say another thing for the entire session, but by that time I felt like no one wanted to deal with my story. I was so frustrated! Then Laura said to me, "You poor kid. You've been keeping this secret from yourself all this time," and then all the feelings came out. Blanche had me sit in Laura's lap. She's very motherly and I like her a lot, and I felt so helpless and impotent, and just cried like a child. Other people in the group comforted me, too—Sam and Miriam and even Charlene, who usually doesn't give a damn about anybody. While I'm getting all this attention, Gloria runs out of the room. Well, too bad.

4 P.M. I have the most incredible conversation with my sister. I tell her about what happened and about the identity of the molester as dear old Uncle Joe, who we always were so afraid of, and now know why, and I ask her whether he abused her, too, and she says, huffily, "He was always very kind to me. But then, you always were the pretty one." I said, "Janet, do you hear what you're saying?" but she said, "Dreams are no evidence. People can dream anything they want. Do you think you're being fair?" and all but hung up on me. What a sick family! What am I to do with all this? I can't handle it!

I went to try to find some place to be alone, and I opened this door and there was Kate, the intake counselor. She invites me in and I start spilling the story about what my sister said and she quietly tells me she was molested by a neighbor when she was seven, that he told her as long as she kept the secret she would be special. "He died, I grieved, and I kept the secret. Then at puberty I found out about sex and that nice girls didn't do it and I began overeating. By my midthirties I was obese and still keeping the secret. Finally I let it go."

I told her I wanted to let it go. I couldn't stand walking around with this information in my head. Kate said I could let go if I forgive him. "Forgive him?" I screamed. "I'll never forgive him. He's practically ruined my life." Kate said forgiveness wasn't for him. It was for me. It was just letting go, and that when I was through processing what I had only just learned this morning, I could let it go and be free. I could be innocent.

I told Kate I've never felt innocent in my whole life, never felt like a child. But today, every now and then, when my mind clears, I feel this still, small voice, clear and pure, and know it's my innocence being heard from at last. It makes me feel clean. I am going to go someplace quiet and listen for it.

9 P.M. The subject at the meeting tonight was pain, and it was astounding to me how few people could feel it. I realized how great this program is because three weeks ago I was just like them. I was doing a lot of nervous laughing and artificial smiling and I was numb. I wish everyone at the meeting could have daily group therapy. These people were all talking in the second person, calling themselves "you" and abstracting, using no examples of their pain, only why they should feel it and how they couldn't. I have compassion for them whereas I found them annoying in the past. I shared for the first time and it felt good. My face felt different as I talked. I felt like I owned my face and voice and they were ageless, sexless, and solid, profound as rock. I felt like my own grandfather.

Day Seventeen
SEXUAL DYSFUNCTION

When people grow up in dysfunctional homes, rarely is their adult sexuality healthy. It has been thwarted along with all their other interpersonal responses. The ability to enjoy sexuality is a clear indicator of a healthy mentality and should be everyone's goal. We are all entitled to enjoy our God-given sexuality without fear or guilt.

Some causes of sexual inadequacy are easy to resolve, such as sexual ignorance, in which case education alone can change a person's values, attitudes, and beliefs. Failure to communicate desires is another problem that can easily be resolved, although many people need to overcome their belief that they don't have a right to experience full sexual pleasure before they can be specific about what they want from their partners. Discord in a relationship can also be the cause of sexual dysfunction, in which case the sexual life of a couple will be adversely affected until they can work out the real problem. Other people use sexuality as a power play, because they feel they have to be in control. They need to learn how to disengage from the power struggle by exploring why they feel they must be in control, and what would happen if they surrendered to the other person. Merely recognizing a power play is going on becomes part of the solution.

Other causes, such as early sexual trauma, are much more difficult to resolve. When children experience a traumatic violation of their boundaries, they have a tremendously difficult time trusting others when they grow up. They are afraid of intimacy and are confused about what it means to get close to someone. They need to learn that intimacy is about shared experiences in the here and now, and that can sometimes but not necessarily include sex.

They also have a lot of trouble enjoying the sexual act. It's hard for them to "be there." If they have repressed their memories of childhood sexual abuse, they must disconnect from what is happening in the present to keep from remembering what happened in the past. Others can give but not experience pleasure in order to maintain their sense of goodness. Whereas some survivors are frigid, letting no one in, others become promiscuous, letting everyone in. Many prostitutes were sexually abused as children.

Sometimes people with a history of childhood sexual abuse indulge in sadomasochistic rituals because they feel a need to be punished for past sins before pleasure can be experienced, or they will create bondage fantasies while having sex. Pretending they are being coerced into the act eliminates the conflict they have over wanting to experience sexual pleasure. Other people who have been sexually abused describe how they jump into threatening and dangerous situations instead of experiencing small pleasures with a "safe" person.

It is also common for these victims of early sexual trauma to sabotage pleasure in other areas of their life. If a job situation or a relationship is going well, something must be wrong. Their fractured sense of reality tells them if they are experiencing pleasure, there must be some kind of sin involved, and for that they must be punished. Often they prefer to self-punish because that way they have some control over how and when it happens, as well as its severity. Self-mutilation is another way they experience a false sense of control over their impulses to self-punish as well as an attempt to reduce anger.

Like food, alcohol, work, or any other source of pleasure, sex can be abused to the point of addiction. It follows the same pattern of progressive self-destructiveness of other addictions, only it masquerades as love. But the sex addict is not really looking for a satisfying relationship. Although that may seem to be the goal, addictive sex objectifies the partner, which makes love and mutual caring an impossibility. The kind of isolation the sex addict feels is perhaps the loneliest of all, because the ritual that brings two people the closest together is for the sex addict a solitary act. Even then he or she is alone, more isolated than ever.

In the early stages of sexual addiction, people use their sexuality to express not love but power, frustration, anger, or as a form of relief from tension or loneliness. Women will have sex when they don't desire it rather than risk losing a relationship, or out of a feeling of obligation. Later on, use escalates to abuse, then progresses to obsession to the point where sex addicts become powerless to control their behavior. In their desperate search for tenderness, they become addicted to the excitement of sexual conquest instead, perpetually on the roam for the next partner.

Sexual addiction takes many forms. For some it becomes complete abstinence, a form of sexual anorexia, or is limited to masturbation. For others it has a binge-and-starve quality: periods of intense activity followed by periods of no activity at all and an overall feeling of numbness. No matter what form it takes, the common denominator is loneliness. Whether acting out or not, the emptiness remains, and the relief experienced has little to do with true bonding.

There are three kinds of 12-step programs for sex addicts, with differing beliefs and aims. The goal of Sex Addicts Anonymous is sexual health and a desire to stop compulsive sexual behavior. Its definition of sobriety does not include abstinence from the sexual act but from "the compulsive, destructive behaviors that rendered our lives unmanageable." Sex and Love Addicts Anonymous deals primarily with self-respect, and its requirement for membership is a desire to stop living out a pattern of sex and love addiction, which it defines as "any sexual or emotional act which, once engaged in, leads to loss of control over rate, frequency or duration of its recurrence, resulting in worsening self-destructive consequences."

Sexaholics Anonymous believes in sexual sobriety and identifies sexual addiction as lust. Its concept of sobriety is the most limiting of the three groups, disallowing any form of sex with oneself or with someone other than a spouse, meaning single people do not indulge in sexual activity.

If you feel a need to belong to a group that addresses problems of addictive sex and love, these groups may be helpful. I find their meetings dignified, and they do not discuss problems in an explicit or offensive way. They are also careful about screening newcomers.

Workbook for Day Seventeen

ASSIGNMENT ONE: SEXUAL VALUES, FEARS, AND PREJUDICES

Complete the following sentences:

1. The way I learned about sex was . . .
2. My most awkward experience with sexuality in adolescence was . . .
3. Watching my parents, I learned . . .
4. My church taught me . . .
5. One of the unspoken messages I got from my mother about me was . . .
6. One of the unspoken messages I got from my father about myself was . . .
7. When I contemplate my mother's impact on my sexual development . . .
8. When I contemplate my father's impact on my sexual development . . .

9. _____ gave me a positive sense of my sexuality.
10. I knew I was a boy/girl when . . .
11. In my family the good thing about being a boy/girl was . . .
12. My first sexual memories are . . .
13. If it turns out I don't need my parents' permission to be a man/woman . . .
14. If it turns out I don't need my parents' permission to be a sexual being . . .
15. If I were fully willing to own and experience my sexuality . . .
16. The most sensual thing is . . .
17. The sexiest thing about me is . . .
18. I like sex when . . .
19. I'm good at sex when . . .

What have you learned about your sexuality from completing these sentences?

A Day in the Life
ELAINE

Wednesday, 9 A.M. Three new people came in today, and I got assigned Kathleen for a buddy. It felt good to take her around and show her everything and reassure her that this place would do her a lot of good. I heard one of them say when she looked over the classroom schedules, "Relationships and sexuality? What's that got to do with dieting?" I just smiled. Some things can't be explained here. It takes a while before you put it all together.

3 P.M. I came from group to find Gloria lying on her bed looking up at the ceiling, and as usual she just ignored me when I asked her what the matter was. Then I went into the bathroom and saw her pile of towels on the floor and decided I had to confront her. I came out and sat on my bed and rehearsed for a few minutes, then said calmly, "You know, Gloria, when you leave towels all over the floor, I feel angry. I need for you to be more respectful of me." Well, the strangest thing happened. She sat up,

stared at me for a while, and then said, "I'm sorry." I couldn't believe it. We started to talk, like two normal people.

Then I was surprised when Jean came in the room and asked Gloria how she was, because they don't get along. At first Gloria was her usual get-out-of-my-face self, but then when Jean ignored that and sat on the bed and said she was sorry for getting so angry at her in group, Gloria started to cry like a little kid. Jean and I sat one on each side of her and held her and tried to get her to talk, but she said she didn't want to talk. She just wanted us to be there and not leave her. Then Blanche knocked on the door and asked for Gloria, and she and Gloria left. Jean stayed. We actually had a conversation. She said she was having a hard time, and I said, "If I can do anything for you, please let me know." Jean said, "When you first came here, I thought you were a phony, but now I really like you." I didn't know what to say. Have I really changed that much? I feel like I'm no one, just a person. Jean told me about how she had come in touch with being molested by her uncle and described her flashbacks and dreams. I told her how I had gotten in touch with an old childhood memory, too, and since then had felt so much more peaceful. Jean said she wished she could feel that, but it's just made her terribly agitated. Later that evening she asked me to sit with her while she phoned her sister, and I did that, but her sister wasn't in. I feel so grateful to be helping others in a real way, not just putting on an act. T think I was even able to touch Gloria in a real way. Something good is happening to me.

Day Eighteen
HEALTHY RELATIONSHIPS

As children, we wanted and deserved unconditional love and didn't get it. Consequently, we keep searching for it, and when it doesn't happen, we work harder at what doesn't work in the first place. As adults we have a choice. We can give and receive mature love. Here are four characteristics of that kind of healthy relationship.

One, it is open to being known to oneself and others.

Both partners are willing to share their feelings and value honesty.

Two, it is accepting of oneself and the differences in others. Can someone take a different route home from the way you go without your getting anxious? Recognize your need for everyone to be the same as you and let it go. Acceptance includes past experiences. They happened. Now, how can they be used to make life better in the present?

Three, the healthy relationship is forgiving of the imperfections in oneself and others. It does not dwell in the guilt and shame of the past or in worry about the future.

Four, the healthy relationship allows for change, in perceptions, attitudes, and behavior. It encourages growth and is not afraid, even of the prospect of growing apart.

An addictive relationship makes a person feel consumed. A healthy relationship allows for individuality. In addictive love there is no definition of ego boundaries. Healthy belonging experiences both oneness with and separateness from a lover. Addictive love exhibits sadomasochism. Healthy loving brings out the best qualities in both partners. Addictive love fears letting go and does not allow for individual growth. Healthy love accepts endings and invites growth in the other partner. Psychological games, giving in order to get, and attempts to change the other are all part of addictive love. In a healthy relationship both giving and receiving are experienced in the same way, and there is no attempt to change or control the other partner.

Addictive lovers feel a need for each other to feel complete. Healthy relationships encourage the self-sufficiency of both partners. The addictive lover demands and expects unconditional love and at the same time refuses commitment. Healthy love is grown-up and does not make infantile demands for unconditional love, and it welcomes commitment as a way of expressing love. Addictive love fears abandonment upon routine separation, looks to the other for affirmation and worth, and desires yet fears closeness. Healthy lovers have a high sense of self-worth, enjoy solitude, welcome closeness, and are able to risk vulnerability. The addictive lover attempts to take care of the other's feelings. Healthy love has boundaries that detach with love.

Mature lovers have conquered the question "Who am I?" They know what they want and need and what is important. In a healthy relationship the partners can appreciate their own individual talents, interests, creative potential, and pursuits. They know their closeness allows for individual difference. Commitment is characterized by desire, not only to give to the other, but to serve the other without expecting something in return. Mature lovers no longer need people in order to survive as they once did in childhood. They are aware that life is harsh at times, unfair at times, and yet continues to be good.

The healthy relationship is close but detached, which means not being distant or *un*involved but being truly grown-up and independent. It means being objective, but not indifferent; flexible, but not indecisive; firm, but not hard; wise, but not clever; patient, but not resigned; strong, but not overbearing; resolute, but not stubborn; compassionate, but not indulgent.

Detachment is profound love, wrapped in understanding and bound by courage. It helps you to live with serenity and fulfillment. It is a goal to strive for, because you deserve it!

Workbook for Day Eighteen

ASSIGNMENT ONE: LETTING GO OF A DESTRUCTIVE RELATIONSHIP

If you are in an unhealthy relationship, or wonder if you are, draw a line down the center of a sheet of paper. At the top of the left-hand column write "What am I losing?" At the top of the right-hand column write "What am I gaining?" Under the left column write down all you are losing, including the qualities you admire in the person you love. Also write down all the qualities you don't admire. For example, maybe you are involved with someone who is a good listener, who is exciting, daring, intelligent, who stands up for what he believes, but is also jealous, blames others for his problems, complains a lot about things he can't change, and does not allow you enough privacy.

Imagine life without this person. What would you gain? Peace of mind? The chance to find a more compatible mate? More personal freedom? Take the time to fully explore your future potential. You might find you *don't* have much to gain from losing this person. If that is so, then maybe you had better reconsider whether this relationship is truly destructive, or whether it can be improved with some help. On the other hand, you might find there is much to gain from letting go of this person, and that may provide you with the resolve you need.

If you have decided you must let go of this relationship, take a look at your list again. The positive aspects you wrote down are the qualities you want to look for in someone else. The negatives are what you want to avoid in someone else. There is never one person on earth for anyone. The world is full of millions of people, many of them engaged in the same search you are. If you seek out the qualities you value, you are likely to find them.

A Day in the Life
TONY

10 A.M. Sam is a great one for telling people he's fine. Mary was in our room and said, "Well, you know what that stands for: Fucked up, Insecure, Neurotic, and Egotistical." Sam thought that was pretty funny and laughed his head off for a while, then said, "I'll never tell anyone I'm fine again." He's a real extreme guy. Bulimics tend to be that way, I've noticed. Jean, too. She's either "never" this or "always" that.

1 P.M. A weird thing happened in group today. Elaine told me I was too bossy. She said whenever she has anything meaningful to say, I cut her off. It surprised me not so much to hear it (because let's face it, I've heard it before) but because it came from Elaine, who is the kind of person who never takes a risk saying something she thinks you might not like to hear. I asked her for an example, and she said that when we were on the bus last

night going to OA, she was telling me about her son and I broke in and started giving her advice she didn't ask for. Smitty asked me how I felt about hearing that, and I just shrugged my shoulders and said, "Okay." He asked others in the group for feedback, but no one wanted to stand up to me I guess. That made me feel worse than hearing what Elaine had to say. Finally this new woman, Leslie, who hasn't had much to say so far, said she thought I was too full of advice, too. I could tell it took a lot out of her to say that. She said I reminded her of her father, and she thought if she took a risk with me it might help her with him. Smitty asked me if Leslie could talk to me about her problems with her father and I said, "Sure." Then Leslie opened up a little bit about feeling out of her element because she was gay and someone had said something about "faggots and queers" on the bus. Smitty kept working on her until she got real angry and started talking about how all her life she had felt like an outsider, missed New York and her community, and was sorry she had come. I told her I didn't have a problem with her being gay and that I wanted to help her. Others started telling her the same, that it didn't make any difference to them, and that they thought she was funny and thoughtful and had a nice smile, etc. She looked relaxed by the time group was over. I hugged her tight and told her she was a great kid.

9 P.M. Leslie knocked on my door. Said she'd been getting up the nerve to do it all night. Pretty soon a bunch of other people were in the room, too. So we're laughing it up and I can tell Leslie's having such a good time she'd rather be with a group than working on her problems with me about her dad. Later for that.

Pretty soon this nurse who has it in for me is poking her head in with her chart wanting to know about bowel movements. She loves to go around asking us whether we had one or not. Leslie pops up, "No, but the night is young." It's amazing to me how there's no embarrassment here about anything, like there's not a damn thing we can do that we have to hide. Crazy. I was glad there were a lot of people in the room and hope they come back tomorrow. I want them on my side when my brother comes down this weekend.

When everybody had gone, I called my wife. I told her I missed her and she started to cry. She said she didn't think I cared about her anymore, and I was shocked. "Where did you get that idea?" I said. "Because you wouldn't sleep with me," she said. I explained to her I had been sleeping in my recliner because I was having a hard time sleeping in bed because I was getting so heavy. "Didn't you know that?" I said. "How should I know?" she wailed. "I thought it was because I only have one breast now." God, that made me feel so horrible. I tried to convince her as best as I could over the phone how much I loved her, more than ever because I had almost lost her and I knew how precious she was, and after we hung up I just shook with anger. After a while I had to get up and walk around. What was I so angry about?

Day Nineteen
ESTABLISHING BOUNDARIES

Boundaries are like a kaleidoscope. They refract the world so you can observe patterns instead of being a victim. I once had a patient who said she couldn't say no to a man under any circumstances. Lacking boundaries to that extent is a form of paralysis. Food, alcohol, and other mood-altering substances create artificial boundaries. Once you abstain from them, you have to learn to create real boundaries in order to feel comfortable in the world.

Boundaries are essential to successful relationships. You can't connect with another unless you are a separate person. Many food addicts come from enmeshed families where members are extensions of each other. If you had thoughts and ideas that were different from those of your relatives, did they feel slighted and offended? If they did, you were not allowed to be separate from them. In such a system, intimacy feels like drowning because your individualism goes down the drain.

People who were not allowed to make boundaries when they were children have a hard time creating them as adults. They guess what others feel, or make people guess what they're feeling. They indulge in magical thinking and endure negative relationships by keeping a fantasy alive that everything is fine.

Creating a boundary means paying attention to your level of discomfort. Addicts are accustomed to all-or-nothing thinking and are not aware of graduals. How close is too close? How much is too much? The only way to determine where those boundaries are is to pay attention to your discomfort level. For instance, if someone is standing too close to you, do you step back? What if that person approaches you again? Will you end up being backed into a corner, or can you say, "When you stand this close to me, I feel uncomfortable"? If you can't make that statement because you don't want the other person to be uncomfortable (although it's all right for you to be!), then you have trouble establishing boundaries.

When people who have difficulty with boundaries do finally manage to establish one and it's crossed, they are really vulnerable. Yet, it's the rare perpetual trespasser who doesn't try, almost as if a boundary line were a challenge. Try not to take it personally. Think of it as a test and pay attention to how you feel. Your discomfort will only increase unless you reestablish your limits.

If the only way you can have a relationship with someone is by tolerating his or her crossing your line, you're not being valued as a person. If you're told "I think you're too sensitive" when you define a boundary, your answer is a resolute "My problem is I haven't been sensitive enough."

You may be surprised at the resistance you will meet when you begin establishing boundaries, especially with those who previously felt free to roam wherever they pleased. For instance, if you tell someone what's important to you and he or she brushes you aside, as if what you said was of no consequence, take note and make a quick exit. This person is not someone to get close to. Or if a person tries to alter what's true for you by saying, "It's really not so bad" or "It's nothing compared to my situation" or "Don't worry about it. Trust me," it's boundary city. My criterion for trust is simply, someone hears what I say and honors it. If I make a statement about myself and someone replies with a statement that begins with

"You should" or "You're too," they've violated my barrier. They can make statements about themselves all they like, but when they make a statement about me, my best interest is in jeopardy.

Assertiveness doesn't guarantee you are correct, or that you will get respect or what you want, but it establishes you as assertive. It sends out the message "Don't tread on me" to those who make a habit of treading on others, deliberately or otherwise. You will recognize who they are when you start paying attention to your body. You will feel discomfort and make a deft getaway.

You are also giving an important message to that little kid you carry around inside—that you are taking care of business, that you matter, that you aren't afraid of a little discomfort to define who you are, and that you don't need the approval of others because you have your own.

People without boundaries are afraid of intimacy because they fear engulfment, for good reason. People keep getting too close, make too many demands. But once you feel safe behind the boundaries you have drawn for yourself, you can establish true intimacy with others.

Workbook for Day Nineteen

ASSIGNMENT ONF

Make a list of your fears. Next to each fear write its opposite. The opposite is what you need. For example, if you fear abandonment, you need closeness. Now make a new list defining what those needs are in detail. Specify alongside each need how you can provide for it. For instance, you may have listed a fear of being alone. Your need is to seek intimacy. You have a fear of poverty. You need a few thousand dollars in a savings account. Be specific.

ASSIGNMENT TWO

Find a partner for this exercise, or better yet, do it with several people. Each person move to a spot in the room where he or she feels safe and comfortable. Then, two by two, begin moving toward one another until your boundaries feel violated. Make eye contact as you do so. As soon as you feel your boundary has been crossed, say so. Have the other person describe the change in your features as the boundary was approached. Ask whether your features changed before you announced your boundary had been crossed, such as frowning, blinking, or involuntary muscle twitching. If you gave indication of discomfort before speaking, you are not paying enough attention to your own discomfort.

ASSIGNMENT THREE

Sit across from a partner. Taking turns, complete the following statements:

"I am willing to . . . I am not willing to . . ."

"I don't wish to do . . . How about . . . ?"

A Day in the Life

JEAN

Friday, 9 A.M. Charlene left last night after two weeks. Her roommate, Laura, is all upset. She thinks there must have been something she could have done to keep her from going, but we all told her she was being her usual co-dependent self. There was nothing and no one who could have kept Charlene from going. She couldn't be talked out of her "my life is wonderful" attitude. Nothing was wrong with Charlene. She just had this strong desire to disappear.

The thing is, I feel awful about not having been able to say something or do something that could have broken through her defenses, too. I know she's not going to make it out there with her overprotective mother and her angry father standing over her all the time demanding that she eat. I bet her mother is waiting for her right now with a big plate of chocolate chip cookies.

10 A.M. Smitty talks about forgiveness. It's a big issue with all us incest survivors. There's a new patient named Bonita who just got in touch with it, and she asks, "But how do I know it really happened? How do I know I'm

not just imagining it?" Smitty says, "Did your parents take you to the top of a mountain and roll you down it in a barrel?" Bonita says, "Of course not." Smitty says, "Because it didn't happen, right? You don't remember things that aren't there to remember. How many people do you know who go around wondering if they were sexually abused? It's just not on anyone's agenda unless it happened. Your mind can lie its head off, but your body never lies. Pay attention to your body and it will tell you the truth."

I have been sitting in circles now for nearly a month and have come to appreciate their value. In a circle you can't hide, you are forced to be a part of the group and participate, even if it is only with body language and eye contact. There is automatic sharing because each person can see and is seen. There is no passivity because there is equality of position. There is more responsibility because no one is hidden. The group is cohesive, linked, and the space in the center is a charged, alive space, a stage for the community agenda. It is much more energetic because each member of the group can more easily contribute and no one is sitting at its head. There is no head.

1 P.M. I totally freaked out in group therapy. I had a confrontation with Gloria and ended up crying hysterically. In spite of all my good intentions I ended up screaming at her and calling her an asshole. I was a complete mess and felt totally unprotected. No one else in group backed me up. They all tell me I acted like a nasty bitch. They tell me in private they think Gloria is a nasty bitch, too, but no one wanted to confront her! I wanted Blanche to tell me Gloria was wrong and I was right, and instead she just let everything be a big mess, even made it worse. "You know, you two are an awful lot alike, and you really have a lot of energy about this. What is it really about?" Blanche wants to know who Gloria really represents for me, but I won't tell her. I didn't think I could get more upset than I already was, but I did when she compared me to Gloria. When I calmed down, I told Blanche she had the same resentful eyes as my sister, and that I just knew Gloria really hated me. Blanche asked me what I needed from Gloria, and I told her I needed her not to storm out when I was talking so I would feel as if she

cares, or not make gestures as if she were going to throw up when I was saying something important the way she did a few days ago.

Blanche wants Gloria and me to explore who we really are for each other. Gloria won't admit I stand for anyone in her life. Then, just as I'm feeling comfortable again, I get hit with being too seductive by Laura, who I thought was my friend! She says my behavior with the men here is inappropriate, and I should check out what it's all about. When Blanche asked others in the group what they felt, I found out they agreed, even Tim! I told him I felt so betrayed, because he's been seductive to me, too! Gloria was really gloating. She says I'm called Scarlett O'Hara. I was so devastated to hear this I wanted to run from the room, but I didn't because that's Gloria's act. I defended myself by saying the older women were just jealous because the men were more attracted to women my age, but Blanche wouldn't let me off the hook. She said I needed to examine why I thought I had to relate to everyone seductively.

Afterward I felt so low I just wanted to check out on the next plane. Instead of going to class I lay on my bed and cried and cried, the most alone I've ever felt in my life. Blanche came looking for me. She has a built-in radar for people in trouble. She asked me if I was ready to fly out of there, but I wouldn't admit it. I told her I want to know my role in conflicts. What do I do that escalates them, and why? What did I say that made me as wrong as Gloria? Could it have been when I called her an asshole? Gee. Blanche says she can feel the pain I'm in, but because she's a codependent she has to let me help myself. She said she really had a hard time holding herself back from helping me. God help me deal with myself! Either take this girl away or let it be neutral! I won't take this. I'm not even going to eat dinner. Everything's too emotionally charged. God, what am I doing? There's a hole in me like a wound poisoning everything. Help me heal, make me better. I feel like it's my group and she invaded. Why are you all letting her yell at me? Why was my sister ever born? It was humiliating like that when Janet and I fought, hating each other, seething silently. I hate my father for preferring her over me! Why can't I let go? I want to die! I know it's true I act seductively with everyone, men and women alike, but I thought I was the only one who knew! It's so hard to deal with the fact that I'm sexually abused and should be sensitive to using sexuality like that. I should be just the opposite and hide it. Not me. Hell, I flaunt it just like it was flaunted in front of me, and that just devastates me.

Day Twenty

STEP STUDY: STEP THREE

"Made a decision to turn our will and our lives over to the care of God as we understood Him."

The first step requires that we acknowledge our powerlessness. The second step requires that we acknowledge a power greater than ourselves. The third step requires more than just acknowledgment. It says we take action; not a small and insignificant action, but make a decision to give away the very things we value the most—our will and our lives! No wonder people balk when they get to this step. Some stay on the threshold of Step Three for years and continue to struggle. That is a painful place to stay in. Others are lucky and surrender their will early, and they are grateful when they experience the Big Surprise, which simply cannot be believed or even comprehended before the step is taken. As soon as we turn our wills over to a power higher than ourselves (and that power need go no further than the power of a 12-step group), we receive more power than we were ever able to give ourselves, a great store of previously untapped resources that we can use for our own benefit and that of others.

If you are still reluctant to relinquish your will, let's examine what your self-sufficiency has done for you. Has it brought you success? Peace of mind? A rich social life? Happiness? Has it fulfilled your goals and set you free of your great craving for food? If it has, you really don't need a 12-step program, and if it hasn't, what are you really giving up?

Do we addicts even possess self-will? If we are in

control of it, why are we so powerless over food? Why can't we put our wills to work for us with enthusiasm? The most enthusiastic people I know, who seem to be tapped into an infinite source of energy, bubbling up in them like a fountain of youth, are very often people who decided to turn their wills and their lives over to God.

When you are ready, Step Three will open the door. In the meantime, you can pray, "Thy will, not mine, be done." God will hear us and give us the serenity we need to take that simple step that seems so impossible from outside the door and so easy once it has been opened. Take a look at the faces of people who have been in a fellowship for any length of time. Do they have the glassy-eyed look of the followers of a secret sect? Or do they seem true to themselves? There is no human being who can be trusted with our will, but we can trust a power greater than ourselves interested only in our living a life that is happy, joyous, and free. We have nothing to lose but our pain.

Workbook for Day Twenty

ASSIGNMENT ONE: GETTING A SPONSOR

Having come this far, you need to find a sponsor. Choose someone with long-term abstinence, someone you heard speak in meetings who inspired you, someone with whom you think you could be completely honest. You are not choosing a friend. You are choosing a bulwark of strength you will be calling every day to "turn over" your food. At the start of each day, you will telephone your sponsor and tell him or her what you plan to eat that day. In doing so, you make a mutual commitment to the program that is reestablished each day. The sponsor is also there to intervene in a slip.

You are not a burden to your sponsor. In fact, sponsors need you as much as you need them, for helping others is necessary to recovery.

Approach the person of your choice and ask him or her to be your sponsor. If that person already has too many sponsees, he or she will help you find another. Take the telephone numbers of other people in meetings, too, and get in the habit of calling people, just to say hello. It is one of the best ways to break your isolation. The telephone is voice-activated reality. Just hearing someone from the program may be all you need to keep from giving in to a self-destructive impulse.

ASSIGNMENT TWO: MEDITATIVE READING: FOOTPRINTS

> One night I dreamed I was walking on the beach with God. In the sky, scenes from my life were flashing, high points of my joy and low points of my suffering. As my path through life flashed across the sky, two sets of footprints marked it in the sand, mine and God's, but to my astonishment, as the saddest and most difficult times were portrayed, only one set of footprints was left below on the sand.
>
> When the last scene from my life passed from the sky, I turned to God and complained, "You said that if I followed you, you'd walk with me all the way, but I can see by the footprints in the sand that you deserted me at the most difficult times in my life. Why did you forsake me when I needed you most?"
>
> And God answered, "My precious child, during the times of your suffering you see only one set of footprints in the sand because it was then that I was carrying you. I have never left you and I never will."

A Day in the Life

ELAINE

Saturday. My family arrives tomorrow and I'm so scared. The family counselors here don't mince words. They really put us on the hot seat and get right down to what our behavior is like with each other, and the group doesn't go lightly either because they really know what's going on—even more than the family counselors do sometimes.

I'm starting to feel really strange about spending time

in a motel room with my husband. I replenished my roommate's body oil last weekend and bought some for myself plus a loofah sponge. Every day now for two weeks I've been scraping off dead skin after my shower and oiling myself, spending more time on the care of my body than I have in years, maybe ever, and my skin is getting so soft and smooth, even my feet. I'm hoping my husband will notice. I'm hoping things will be different between us now sexually, but don't know what to expect. I talked about it in group yesterday (I'm getting so brave I amaze myself), and Smitty said, "Why don't you just wait and get yourself surprised?" I thought that was good advice! I feel like a virgin. Maybe I am.

11 P.M. We had a dance here in the dining room. We turned on a local radio station and Tony flashed the light switch on and off real fast like a strobe. I even danced. It's great to see people getting out of their depression and shaking it. I love everyone here. T.J. and one of the other nurses on duty tonight secretly called the radio station and suddenly the DJ said, "Hey, keep it cool up there on the second floor of a certain hospital." It was uproarious. Jean says, "Can I stay here forever?" Every now and then I would get waves of bad feelings that all this fun was not allowed, but I would not give in to them. Now I'm reading in bed and I hear laughter in the hall, clapping, hoots, and applause, people coming out of their shells with a vengeance. I want to get some sleep, though. Tomorrow's going to be a big day.

Day Twenty-one
UNFINISHED BUSINESS

It's hard to look down to the bottom of a well and see what's there. People with unfinished business from their past must be brave enough to beam a strong light into the depths, acknowledge what they find, experience the pain of it, and then express that pain. It's a shame to be hurting today for something that happened to you a long time ago.

If you have spent a lifetime suffering from old and painful memories, or spend a lot of time whistling in the dark to mask the sound of monsters rustling behind closet doors you won't open, you must get out of the poisonous environment you're in. However, entropy must be taken into consideration. Until you take a good look at what happened and truly feel it, you won't move on to a better place.

Anger, fear, grief, guilt, shame, resentment, and other painful feelings are negative energy, and that energy needs to be charged and disposed of in a safe place so you can get on with your life. If you have been carrying around feelings you have never expressed surrounding childhood abuse, it's time you get rid of them.

In group therapy unfinished business is called anger work, and it is highly structured because the experience can be frightening, and you may feel completely out of control. Ground rules are carefully laid beforehand so participants know what to expect. Here is a typical example: A person has been working hard in group for several weeks, bringing up long-submerged anger at an abusive parent. He has been told to write a letter to that parent and bring it to group. While he reads it, the feelings he suppressed as a child surface and begin to overwhelm him. He is ready to re-create the painful memory and express the rage and grief he has never felt safe enough to experience.

The therapist puts an empty chair in front of him, a substantial chair that will quite literally take a beating, and the patient is given a pillow. There is only one rule: He must not hurt himself or others when he expresses his anger. For instance, he can beat the pillow with an open hand but not with a closed fist because that might hurt his hand and he has been hurt enough. He can hold the pillow in his fists and beat the chair. He can cry and rage and beat out his anger until it is gone. Sometimes more memories come up in the process of expressing anger, more pain and grief, and they, too, are acknowledged and expressed. The others in the group are there for him completely. They comfort him and validate his experience. They tell him how they have drawn strength from his courage. They hold him afterward and allow him to fully express his grief.

The power of the energy of anger is awesome, particularly in those who have never allowed themselves to tap into it. After the event, people often sleep. They wake feeling purged, as if they had lost weight, for they have. They have lost the heavy burden of unexpressed emotions they have carried all their lives. They now are free to travel light, minus the burden of the past. Taking care of unfinished business often results in permanent change: once you take your trash to the dump, you don't have a yen to go back for it afterward. The same is true for these toxic feelings: When they're gone, they're gone.

Unfinished business is not limited to people with issues of childhood abuse. People who suffered from neglect as children often have a much more difficult time getting in touch with anger. The abuse victim has some traumatic memory to find, but the victim of neglect has only a vague and amorphous nothingness. They can't point to any scars. The abuse victim has flashbacks or self-mutilates, or has memories of being hit or verbally assaulted. Victims of neglect have no picture of what they missed and no sense of what they need. If they've done without, they have no reason to think they're worthy. Neglect is the climate they lived in, and its all-pervasive and undramatic nature is difficult to focus on.

Survivors of neglect often say, "My greatest fear is I *have* no problems." When they seek their inner child, they often find it hiding, or can't find it at all. "I ran away from home once when I was little," a victim of neglect once told me, "and when I came back, I found no one even knew I was gone." The neglect victim is often the slowest to bring up anger and grief that needs to be expressed in order to feel again. In group they are reluctant to have attention focused on themselves because their problems are so "insignificant, no big deal." "Other people have real problems," they will tell you, "I'm just neurotic."

The same difficulty is true for those who suffered religious abuse as children. It's a lot less threatening for people to bring up an abusive parent than an angry, jealous deity who has the power to read their thoughts and strike them dead! You can run away from an abusive parent, but how do you escape from an all-powerful God who can punish you for eternity?

The combined authority of parents and clergy may be too threatening to challenge, even in a safe therapeutic environment, and may be buried so deep that all that can be seen are the symptoms: human beings who cannot enjoy the simple pleasures of life, the right to live free of guilt, and to experience their own sexuality. People who suffered from religious abuse need to put that punishing "God" in the chair and go at *him* with a pillow. Afterward they find they have room for a loving God, who will help them learn to be happy, joyous, and free as we were put on this earth to be.

Sometimes unfinished business is not so traumatic. It might be a recent or a past ungrieved-for loss. I have seen people in treatment weep for lost pets from their childhood and have been moved to tears at their outpouring of grief. It doesn't matter what the cause of the unfinished business is as much as that it has never been acknowledged, experienced, or expressed. Your reaction to reading this will confirm for you the kind of unfinished business you may have to take care of. You may have little or no reaction to it, but if you are agitated and full of negative feelings right now, my bet is you've got some bottled-up righteous anger in you that needs to be uncorked. If you want to recover, you must take care of your unfinished business. Make it your number-one priority, for you deserve to live fully. Seek help.

Workbook for Day Twenty-one

ASSIGNMENT ONE

If you are in group therapy and feel you are ready to deal with your unfinished business, discuss it with your therapist. You may want to write a letter to the person or persons whom you have never confronted about hurtful events that occurred in your childhood that are still making you unhappy today. You may never need to confront them. The anger work is for yourself, so you can feel better. It will set you free from the prison of your past.

ASSIGNMENT TWO: YOU ARE A CELEBRATION OF LIFE!

Affirmation for a Troubled Mind

I know the quality of what I have
and it cannot be devalued
I know the source of all my strength
and have tapped into its power
I know the beauty of my soul
and that it can't be altered
I know I am God's child
I know I am God's child.

I know I am a treasure and my preciousness is
real
I know these feelings in me now are only
passing through
I know that it's my right to be joyous and be
free
And I know I am God's child
I know I am God's child.

I feel the power of a love that is constant and all
giving
I feel the pull to goodness within me even now
I feel your strength embrace me as I tremble in
this time
I can comfort my own child
I can comfort my own child.

A Day in the Life

TONY

Sunday, 1 P.M. I have to write about this incredible thing that happened the other day in group. I've been processing it ever since and want to write it down to try and clarify it. I brought up the conversation I had with my wife the other night and how bad I felt about her thinking I didn't want to sleep with her because of her mastectomy, and how angry I had been feeling ever since, and Smitty kept at me about where the anger was coming from until suddenly I realized I was angry at her cancer. So fucking angry at the cancer! I had never realized how angry I had been at that. Was it crazy to be angry at a disease? Instead of answering me Smitty gets this look in his eye and I think, oh-oh, he's going to want me to do anger work and there's no way I'm going to pound a pillow. I'm too afraid of my anger to do that, too afraid I'd kill the chair if I really let loose. Instead he hands me the yellow pages and tells me, "This is your wife's cancer. What do you want to tell it?" I'm holding the yellow pages in my hands, thinking how angry I was, and suddenly there was only one thing to do, and a white-hot light went through me, just like a flash of lightning, and I felt myself ripping the yellow pages clean in half, right down the middle, slowly, purposefully, with more power than I knew I had, and it felt so good, so powerfully good. Afterward everybody just sat there. I was grinning like hell. I mean, I ripped that fucking phone book neatly in half! "Look at his face," Smitty said. Elaine said, "You look like a boy." Others agreed. It was as if taking my anger out on that phone book had dropped ten or twenty years off me. I was sore in my arms and shoulders for hours afterward. The force it took was much greater than I realized at the time.

That night of course I had to call my wife and tell her. She says, "I've got to see that phone book before I'll believe it." I got out of bed and went into the room where we have group and sure enough, Smitty saved it. Afterward when he asked me what I wanted to do with the two pieces of the phone book, I had sort of cavalierly thrown them in the wastebasket as if it were nothing, but he had retrieved them and put them on a shelf. So now they're in my room.

The funny thing is, I'm in a different place since that happened. I feel so full of energy, and so full of love for everyone here, even Gloria. The other day when I said, "How're you doing?" and she said, "Buzz off!" I just laughed and said, "I know you don't mean that." She ran out of the room and I knew it was because it was all she knew how to do. Poor kid. I wonder what her trouble is.

Elaine's husband, son, and daughter just arrived. They're in having group with Smitty. I have this scary feeling in the pit of my stomach, knowing my brother is coming tomorrow night and I'll be having to deal with him. Elaine was a nervous wreck going in there. Her husband seems like a real nice guy, obviously loves her a lot. Her kids look sort of dazed. I was surprised to see her daughter was really fat. Elaine has never mentioned that.

Just as I was feeling really down, people started coming into my room. It's gotten to be like the main gathering spot since Sam arrived. He's a good-looking guy, tall and muscular and full of manic energy. I couldn't believe what he pulled. There were four of us in here, Mary, Leslie, Sam, and me, when we heard the bell that means the dinner carts have arrived, the ones I used to lurk around the elevators waiting for. Sam jumped up, and the next thing I knew, he was rolling a whole cart in here, trays stacked ten high, and saying, "Let's binge!" Mary pulls herself together and rolls the trays back in the hall before anyone notices.

7

Week Four

On the Path to a New Life

Behavioralists say it takes twenty-one days to establish a new habit. You have now passed that mark. Your new routines are no longer a totally conscious effort, and you are beginning to feel serene about this new direction you've taken. The struggle is beginning to diminish between the forces within you that want to go back to the old way and the new forces that want to take you another, but every now and then you still feel caught in the pull. Every now and then the addict in you is going to come out for a noonday stroll. You will know when it's out because you will feel the loss of serenity.

Twenty-one days of abstinence from white flour, sugar, and caffeine is now beginning to show—in your eyes, the rosy glow of your complexion, in the open and relaxed look of your face—and others are beginning to remark on it. Twenty-one days of daily exercise is making you strong. Even when your mind feels sluggish, your body is raring to go, and you find you want to do more. Follow the urge and enroll in an exercise program, but keep up the daily walk.

Your affirmations are resulting in a new attitude that is also being acknowledged by others. Your positive outlook and humor are attracting them. Whenever you receive a compliment, don't reject it. Rub it in! You deserve it, don't you think? You are now in a feedback loop that will work to increase your motivation. Congratulate yourself for the days you spent in commitment to this program without any positive feedback. Now you can reap the benefits of that blind faith you exhibited the first few weeks.

Week Four is about reaping what you have so diligently and sometimes painfully sowed. Suddenly everything seems possible. Believe me, it is, and more at this point than you can even imagine.

Day Twenty-two

SAY WHAT YOU MEAN, MEAN WHAT YOU SAY, BUT DON'T SAY IT MEAN!

If you don't allow yourself to express feelings, they grow until you finally explode. That's appropriate for anger work, but not for the feelings you have that are connected to the present. If you want to stop acting like a victim, you need to learn how to express your feelings in spite of the fear you feel. Not expressing them may give you some short-term relief, but it will result in long-term pain that will escalate until you are unable to express them in a way that will get you what you want. The victim acts out; the survivor takes action. The victim reacts; the survivor responds. Today we will be concerned with the two sides of effective communication: good listening and assertive expression of feelings and needs.

The goal of listening is understanding. It is the best gift you can give to anyone, and perhaps the best way to communicate love and respect.

The Listening Ladder

L: Look at the person speaking
A: Ask questions for clarification
D: Don't change the subject
D: Don't interrupt
E: Express emotions with control
R: Responsibility to listen

You, as a good listener, look into the eyes of whoever is speaking and see them for who they are today, not someone they remind you of. You devote your energy to taking in what they have to say, withholding evaluation of the message and not judging it or overreacting to it. The good listener in you does not interrupt or change the subject, but when feedback is requested, you will give it, clearly and sincerely. You are tolerant and don't let a person's manner of speaking turn you off. You concentrate on facts but listen for the feelings behind what is being said, and you don't let emotion-arousing words disrupt the listening process. If someone is having difficulty expressing emotion, lean back. If someone is really desperate to be heard, lean forward. Responsibility for listening also means letting people know if you don't have time to listen rather than faking attentiveness.

Good listening takes energy and discipline. If you are a good listener to yourself, you will be a good listener to others. When you respond to someone who's in need of being understood, keep the focus on the other person rather than saying, "I know how you feel. A similar thing happened to me . . ." You invalidate someone's uniqueness when you compare their experiences to your own. Instead, ask questions that will result in the speaker's telling you more, such as, "I don't understand what you mean by . . . ," "I'm glad you . . . ," or touch them in a way that conveys your understanding.

When the situation is reversed, you can become a

more conscious communicator. When calling someone on the telephone, you can say, "Do you have a few minutes? I really need to talk," rather than barging in with your problem.

When you really want to communicate with someone, ask for what you need. Most likely you have trouble doing that, or even knowing what it is you need because you put a low value on giving yourself what you readily give to others. As we learned last week, the best way to discover what you need is to look at what you fear, which is usually more readily identifiable. Once you identify your fears, you can know what your needs are, because they are the opposite of your fears. If you fear rejection, you need acceptance. If you fear being controlled, you need autonomy. If you fear abandonment, you need belonging. If you fear being abused, you need nurturance.

F—False
E—Evidence
A—Appearing
R—Real

You have two choices: fear with action or fear with no action. Choose fear with action because it keeps you moving, whereas fear with no action bogs you down. Fear is never going to leave your life. It's an emotion like love or sadness. You're not doing anything wrong if you're afraid. It's the inaction that's debilitating.

The more you operate out of fear, the greater the likelihood that your fears will come true, for the mind tends to move toward its most dominant thought. The greater your fear of rejection, the more likely you will be rejected and reject others before they have a chance to reject you. If instead you honor your need for acceptance, learn to ask for it, and create situations in which it will likely come about, your needs will take precedence over your fears. Like two ends of a seesaw, the higher the need reaches toward fulfillment, the lower the fear recedes.

You may feel foolish at first asking for what you need, but you will find it disarms people because it is nonconfrontational. It makes you human, because you acknowledge you have needs and are willing to expose your vulnerability. Needs can't be denied, rejected, or argued about. They are a solid basis for honest communication.

Workbook for Day Twenty-two

ASSIGNMENT ONE: LISTENING

With your buddy take turns speaking for three minutes about something that is bothering you. Choose who will speak first. Sit close together and look into each other's eyes. While one is talking, the other listens and *does not verbalize* but finds nonverbal ways to respond to what is being said. Let silences go by, and allow the one who is talking to think without the listener feeling obligated to fill the silence. After three minutes, change roles.

This listening exercise will show you how powerful an advocate you can be by saying nothing. It may also show you how difficult it is not to respond when someone else is talking. Let the discomfort be your guide as to where you need to work on your communication skills.

A Day in the Life

JEAN

Monday, 10 A.M. I just got a telephone call from my sister. She said she wants to come see me. I was really surprised, seeing as how she practically hung up on me when I told her about my flashbacks, and I asked her what had changed her mind. At first she said she didn't want to talk about it on the phone, but finally I convinced her to tell me. She said she had been thinking a lot about what I had said, and she had more or less hung up on me because she had never been able to face the fact that what Uncle Joe had done to her was sexual abuse. She started to break down then, and I realized with a shock that I had never heard her really cry. I tried to help her by telling her the things I've learned here about incest, such as how the victims carry the guilt and shame and how we've got to stop doing that. She said he had always told her she was special, and said she was jealous and upset that he had told me the same thing. I told her how much I appreciated her honesty and how close it made me feel to her.

Then she really got upset. "But that's not why I'm calling. That's history. I asked Patti if Uncle Joe had done something to her when we were home. I told you how she's been acting strange, falling asleep in school because she can't sleep at night, and oh, Jeannie, he's been abusing her, too. That sick bastard! I could kill him!" I told her to hang on and ran and got Blanche, who listened to her for a long time and then gently and firmly told her to come in for counseling as soon as she could arrange it. When she got off the phone, I said, "But what about my parents? This is going to make so much trouble! Uncle Joe is my mother's favorite brother! Dad is going to want to kill him! But wait, they might not even believe us! What if they get mad and tell us we're making the whole thing up?" Blanche said to put the matter on the shelf until my sister arrives. Until then I can concentrate on what this has done to me. The horrible feelings I'm having about my niece are the same feelings I should be having for myself. I was the same helpless, innocent little girl then that she is now. It's just easier to feel sorry for my niece than feel anything for myself.

I'm so glad my sister and I don't have to handle this all by ourselves. We all would have suffered in silence, into a second generation now, if it hadn't been for this place. I feel so close to my sister. Maybe we can finally drop our defenses and stop being so competitive, now that we know the sick origins of that competitiveness. Suddenly this whole thing is giving me a giant headache. Blanche is right. I can't solve this problem today.

1 P.M. Group. My developing friendship with Gloria helps me understand myself. Today Blanche said to her, "Gloria, why is it I can't make a connection with you? I've been trying for three weeks to get you to see how much I care, and it seems like nothing's happening." For some reason, that did it. Blanche connected. Gloria just melted into a little girl, with a vulnerable little girl's stance and voice, and then she really let loose and belted the empty chair with the pillow, yelling at her father until she collapsed. Then Blanche played some soothing music and each woman in the group held Gloria in her arms, rocking

her gently back and forth and whispering in her ear that we loved her and she was going to be all right. At first Gloria got all tight, as if she couldn't breathe, but then she just sighed, as if she were all worn-out, and allowed us to care for her. Afterward, Gloria told me that I was her inspiration. Because I had allowed myself to bring out what had happened to me, to go dig for the memory and not let go of it, she decided she couldn't continue to block out what she knew was happening and continued to happen. Instead of going home to deal with more abuse, she's going to a halfway house, get a job, and decide what she's going to do with her life. She's so brave, and only nineteen. If she can do it, I can do it, too.

8 P.M. I relapsed. I went into the bathroom, stuck two fingers down my throat, and threw up.

Day Twenty-three
FORGIVENESS

Forgiveness does not require that you tell the people who did you harm that you are forgiving them. It is a selfish act done only for yourself so you can feel better. In no way does it condone what they did. Rather, it is a conscious decision to surrender your feelings. Anger, resentment, and hate are luxuries we food addicts can't afford, for they will cause us to relapse back into our addiction.

Forgiveness is a release of feelings: you must feel them, deal with them, and give them up, so the space they took up can be filled with love. You don't have to forgive everyone at once, only as you can. When you want hate less than love, you will be willing to make the exchange.

Forgiveness is the key to loving yourself. If you can choose not to forgive and hold on to your pain, you can also choose to let go, for there are two sides to everything. Mary A. Dombroski, Ph.D., has developed a helpful acronym for the forgiveness process called ADDS:

> *Awareness* means crossing the threshold of denial and acknowledging the wrongs inflicted happened and that they hurt.
>
> *Discovering* means sharing those feelings

> with others, for communicating them makes them real. You have been carrying the burden of your secret, and sharing that secret does away with it just as a sunrise does away with night. Once a secret is shared, it loses its power and becomes real.
>
> *Decision* means a willingness to let go. Holding on to the discovery will give it power again. Detaching from it is a choice to make for health.
>
> *Serenity* is the healing gift of forgiveness.

When people don't forgive, it's about false pride and being judgmental. Humility is about forgiving. It's learning to come to everyone with love, even people who have wronged you. It doesn't matter what people do. It's more important what you do. I know it hurts and I'm not negating the emotional or physical pain if you've been injured by someone, but I think to have dignity we have to come to everyone out of love. That's why forgiveness is so important. Without it you can't come from love.

Workbook for Day Twenty-three

ASSIGNMENT ONE

Draw up a list of three people who have hurt you. Write each one a letter, describing in detail the harm they did to you and how it has affected your life. Describe the feelings you still carry about their deeds. Take each letter, crumble it in a ball, put it in a sink, and set fire to it. As it burns, say, "I forgive you." When the letters are nothing but ashes, dispose of them, clean the sink, and get on with the business of living.

ASSIGNMENT TWO: VISUALIZATION FOR FORGIVENESS

Sit comfortably and quiet your mind as you have been practicing. One by one, visualize the people who harmed you as a child as little children themselves. Focus on their faces and note whether they are sad. If they are, ask them what they need. Then reach in and embrace those little children. Tell them that you love them and are setting them free.

A Day in the Life
ELAINE

Tuesday, 10 A.M. My children are talking quietly in the next room as I write this. I am so comforted by the sound. It was painful in family therapy with Smitty to hear the stark reality of their childhoods as they described how I wasn't there for them. I have only recently come in contact with my own pain, and it's the same as theirs, being lonely in the presence of others. I know what they meant when they said that even though I was always there—busy making a nice home, cooking nutritious meals, on every parent committee at school, driving them to their music lessons, and waiting with them at the orthodontist—I was always so aloof, so cheerfully *not there*.

I didn't beat up on myself about it, though. I shared with them that I understood what they meant about my not being at home, and I told them it was only recently that I had made my own acquaintance myself. We all had a good laugh about that. It filled me with such relief to acknowledge the truth. We sat in a circle around Smitty and the tears just couldn't stop flowing. Even my husband cried. As I sat there thinking about how I wished things could have been different for my kids, how I wish I could have spared them this loneliness, my parents flashed across my mind. Those poor people couldn't give what they hadn't been given either, and in a rush of love I forgave them. Now the tears that flowed were tears of healing. I want to hold on to that feeling of forgiveness. Hate has nowhere to go.

This morning while it was still dark, I nudged my husband and we went out on our motel balcony and watched the sunrise. It was an incredible production, pink and blue and lemon flashes illuminating the clouds before the sun even appeared. We watched until the light glowed on the tree trunks across the parking lot, standing for a long time with our arms around each other. I felt such peaceful joy, and I let it flood my whole being like the sun had just flooded the earth with the most gloriously colored light. We went back into our room. Without a word I started undressing him, then stood perfectly still while he undressed me, murmuring words of appreciation, which I now choose to believe. I am not my body, I am me, and I am all right. In fact, I'm wonderful, just as he's been trying to tell me for years.

I've never really known arousal before. I've never even liked making love unless it's completely dark. Yet, here we were in the morning, like newlyweds after a night of passion, going at it again—at my instigation! My husband can't get over these changes in me and neither can I. When I confessed I had been faking orgasms all these years, he said he knew, and didn't I think I had a lot of lost pleasure to make up for? Please understand we've never had such a discussion in our entire marriage—or rather he has, but I would get all nervous and tell him to stop, that I didn't want to hear about it, that some women were just naturally frigid. Well, this morning, lo and behold, I found out I'm not. What a surprise, to find out my own body is the source of so much fun! No wonder everyone's so keen on making love. I truly did not get the message, and I am so grateful I have the rest of my life to make it up to myself. And to my husband, too.

Day Twenty-four
THE "REAL YOU" EMERGES

You are what you are what you are, if you can just step out of your way. With enough letting go, that positive and creative human being will be set free. In the course of treatment, you have let go of the defense mechanisms you had been using to protect your real self, letting go on faith that you were doing the right thing. You have let go of your past and reframed your early childhood messages, acting to change them instead of struggling with them. You have let go of the roles you play in lieu of who you really are. You have let go of grief and loss of love from the past, allowing negative emotions to surface, and you have accepted your limitations, letting go of the need for perfection and your magical thinking. You have let go of your family and personal secrets and practiced forgiveness. You have identified painful underlying issues, taken care of unfinished business, and allowed yourself to be helpless and powerless, vulnerable and without defenses.

You have let go of your isolation and begun to bond with others, and you have practiced relaxation techniques to reduce stress and fear. You have taken risks by acting assertively and expressed feelings in effective and appropriate ways. You have made choices in spite of your fears and built trust in yourself and others. You have established boundaries and defended them, learning communications skills that allow you to say what you mean and mean what you say, to respond instead of react, and to share instead of tell. You have developed healthy eating patterns and rituals to change your negative thought patterns to positive ones. You have learned to hug, laugh, and feel. You have become real, and in the end, that is all that matters.

You have become a spiritual being, translucent, open, someone who lives in the here and now, who dares to be spontaneous, who is glad to help others. You know you are not your body but God's child, and you love who that is. You love who you are and want to claim your power. You're confident. You respond, not react, and that empowers the Real Me.

Love does not fail you when you don't get it. It fails you when you don't give it. Love does not guarantee popularity. Love requires that I say what I believe and do what I consider right. As addicts, we demand love and treat people or allow others to treat us as things—objects for love. But real love allows people room to breathe, to have their own identity, to be responsible for themselves, sometimes loving the person enough to let go.

Real love is passion, commitment, and intimacy. Passion is the powerful force in nature that draws two people together for procreation, but it will not last beyond a few days or weeks if that is all there is to the connection. Commitment is also necessary, the glue that keeps a relationship going after the initial excitement is over. But people sometimes stay together out of commitment alone, without experiencing real love. That needs a third element, intimacy. As you have learned, you can't be intimate with another until you know and love yourself. You are now ready for real love. You can choose whom you will become intimate with rather than settle out of fear and desperation. Your repressed sexuality, sensuality, and creativity will start to flow, and you will become exciting to others.

Father Booth likes to draw a triangle to show what true spirituality is. One side is emotions, the second body, the third mind, all encompassed in Spirit. He disagrees with the concept that the human being is mind, body, and spirit, and so do I, for it isolates spirituality from body and mind. Especially in dealing with eating disorders and its abuse of the body, it's important that people start to love and take care of their bodies as a spiritual entity. The sum of all our parts is our spirituality. God lives in us and other people in a state of tangibility. This kind of spirituality couldn't be further from the kind of religion that imprisons the spirit, that molests people's minds with ideas that sex is dirty, that menstruation is "the curse," that you can't go to God without a priest, that everything we enjoy, God is against. It's staggering how many obese people attend these religious centers where spirituality is abused.

I believe you become like the God you believe in, so if you believe in a God of anger, you'll be angry, in a God who judges, you'll judge. But if your God is loving, accepting, and caring, you will become those things, too.

Workbook for Day Twenty-four

ASSIGNMENT ONE: BODY IMAGE

Ask yourself:

1. Whose body would you most want yours to look like? Why?

2. How do you feel about your body? What features do you like best about yourself? What features do you like least?

3. Close your eyes and take time to create scenes of yourself in the body you would like to have in the following situations—an office party, playing volleyball at a picnic, having sex. How would you move, talk, and envision others seeing you? See how you interact with the opposite sex.

ASSIGNMENT TWO

(To be done with your buddy.) Gift Box: Six gifts from your Higher Power. Into six envelopes put the following six messages:

1. A profound ability to make contact.
2. An extraordinary collection of feelings, all of them good.
3. The magical ability to laugh, dance, and sing.
4. The magical ability to nurture and heal another.
5. A sacred capacity to forgive.
6. The ability to rest luxuriously.

One person at a time opens all six envelopes, expresses joy at the gift, and describes how it will be used.

Enjoy life. This is not a dress rehearsal!

A Day in the Life
TONY

Wednesday, 11 A.M. I felt terrific Monday sitting up in front with Elaine, Jean, and Gloria at commencement, looking out on the new arrivals, their confusion and denial a mirror of what I was nearly four weeks ago. We spent hours composing this poem and then elected Gloria to recite it:

The first day was terrible—hysteria and fear
What is this commencement? Do people really
leave here?
Confusion, upheaval, no room at the Inn
Here a pill, there an oat bran, it seems like a
no-win.

Then came group sessions, all screaming and
tears
Confrontive, confrontive, let's uncover those
fears!
Sadness, madness, anger, pain
All these emotions came down like the rain.
Pushed by the counselors, homesick as hell
But also new friendships which bonded us well.
Walk out those tensions, but always in two's
Roommates to talk to, to chase away blues.
The third week was quiet, thoughtful and
pensive
A new spark inside. I won't be submissive.
Time for the bus again, everyone here?
Bumpitty bump—move over, dear.
OA, AA, NA, ACOA
You can use your change but get the right kind
of soda.
Mile after mile we travel our way
So many issues to unravel today.
But there's Rosalie and Smitty with a helping
hand
Blanche and Vickie find a soft place to land.
The nurses that watch us—"Turn your back to
the scale!"
Then there's Tim with his stares and weekends
with Sal.
The last week is here, anticipation begins
But now I am strong and I know I will win.
I'm loving and trusting—hopeful and proud
I'm excited and joyful—even laughing out loud!
Now we gather, to say good-bye to all
I feel grateful and thinner—I'll follow the call.
Some pain and fear stays here, I leave behind
the strife
But what travels away *is* a celebration of life.
Freedom at last, the ties that bind are gone
My soul is connected and the burden has flown
The tools are in my Big Book, my eyes can
clearly see
All I ever needed—how simple—is here
inside of me.

My brother Robert arrived late last night. He had a hundred excuses why he was two days overdue, but I didn't mind. I was kind of hoping he wouldn't come. We had a session with Smitty that was really rough. It seems Robert has been scared of me all his life, even though he's the older brother. I told him I felt he had all the advantages—smarter, more attractive to the women, better at sports—I had to act feisty to hold my own. We did a lot of yelling at each other at first, and Smitty just sat there and let everything be a mess. Finally we both piped down a bit and I even apologized. I said I was learning how to express myself without getting angry all the time. Robert said he was far from perfect himself, that he knew he had let me shoulder too much of the burden in the family as well as in the business, but every time he tried to help I gave him a strong message that I could do it better. "Maybe you can, Tony," he said, and I felt so bad. I told him it was too much of a burden for one person, and that I needed him. I'll be damned if he didn't get out his handkerchief and pretend to wipe his brow, but I knew he was wiping away tears in the process. Then he blew his nose real loud. "I want to be needed," he said. "I know I haven't always acted responsibly, but I can learn."

We embraced. I still don't trust him, but I'll try like hell to.

9 P.M. We went to an OA meeting together, and I shared for the first time. I thought it was going to be so hard, but it wasn't. The words came from somewhere. I told how I knew I had a problem when I ordered the shopping bag full of Chinese food and didn't remember eating it afterward. I told how I could control my business, my home, my finances, my family situation, my friendships, but I couldn't control a salami sandwich. That got a laugh. I told how my first ten days in treatment I had my bags packed and was ready to go, that I really believed I'd made a big mistake coming here, and the trouble I had with all the God stuff, and then how everything started to come together in the last four or five days but I couldn't explain it. Everybody was smiling at me as if I didn't need to explain anything, that my standing before them was all the explanation they needed. I sat

down and my brother put his arm around my shoulder. That did it. The tears came. I didn't even care if he saw.

Day Twenty-five
WINNING PERSONALITIES

The first quality of winning is so important—the quality of self-esteem, knowing you deserve to win. There never was a winner who didn't feel that he or she deserved to win. *It's not really pride in what you've done or what you have; it's the deep-down, inside-the-skin feeling of your own worth.*

Positive self-esteem is the single most important human quality in a salesman, manager, leader, mother, father, or child. It is the feeling that I accept and believe in myself as a changing, imperfect, growing human being. Pride is based on what you have or have done. Self-esteem is based on what you are going to do and what you feel you deserve. I see people holding back because they don't want the loneliness that comes with distancing when you are a winner, but they don't see that farther down toward the finish line there's plenty of company—in the winner's circle.

Remember, you always move toward your dominant thought—every minute of every day. You can't move away from what you're thinking. You move toward your fears just as if they were your goals. You can't dwell on the reverse of an idea. If you're going to motivate your children, your employees, your friends, and yourself, tell yourself what you want and move yourself in the direction of your winning thoughts.

Positive self-motivation is an inner drive, a dissatisfaction with the status quo, a desire for change. It takes place in two prominent emotions: fear in the negative and desire in the affirmative. Fear is the greatest motivator of all, telling you that you have compulsion, which is "have to." Fear is the greatest red light in the world telling you that you can't, which is inhibition. Fear is the strongest compeller and the strongest inhibitor.

Desire is 180 degrees apart and is the greatest propeller. If fear is a compeller, desire is a propeller. Motivation is movement or action toward the current dominant motive.

The winner focuses the intensity on the desired result. You must always focus your intense thought on the reward of success and where you want to go. You cannot look back, you must look at the focus of the result.

Be willing to dream—to have clearly in mind what it is you want. The mind is the most magnificent biocomputer ever created. It doesn't relate to getting through the day or being happy, or other general ideas. Winners dream about their goals. They dream specifically with words, pictures, and emotions.

Positive self-direction is focusing on a purpose. If you don't have a purpose, your system will set one for you—to get through the day. It will give you just enough energy to watch TV. The most important thing I've ever found is that if you plan to fail, then fail to plan, and beginning is half done. Beginning anything is half done.

Of all the things I know, purpose is the key. People die on purpose, and people die because of no purpose. I heard of a famous personality's saying to his daughter, "I'm tired now, I'm going to do nothing for the rest of my life." He was dead in nine hours. There are two great tragedies in life—never to have had a target and never to have reached it. Reaching your target is up to you.

Goals and dreams need to be internalized. A major key to winning is the internalization of goals, which is known as simulation or self-discipline. Perhaps more than any other characteristic of a winner, the ability to "practice within when you're without" is the key to winning. The imagination is the most powerful tool of all. Winners realize that in your imagination you never have to miss. Every salesperson closes the sale in advance. Every host or hostess plans the party in advance. Winners practice in their imaginations—over and over simulating the winning experience. *Winners in life have persistence. They hang in there.*

Here are some winners to emulate:

Helen Keller. Winning is a blind and deaf girl who devoted her life to the less fortunate.

Albert Einstein. Winning is the high school boy who

failed his college entrance exams and went on to develop the theory of relativity.

Wilma Rudolph. Winning is the little girl who had a siege of double pneumonia and scarlet fever, didn't walk without leg braces until she was eight, and yet went on to become the fastest woman in the world, winning four gold medals in the 1960 Olympics.

Abraham Lincoln. Winning is the man who failed in business, lost his sweetheart, failed at public office eight times, and yet went on to become one of the most beloved of our presidents.

Winners do things for the benefit of others rather than at their expense. They relate to the world around them in a positive way. They have the most important quality of all—dimension. Dimension is perspective. It is the ability to plant a shade tree under which you know you'll never sit. It is the ability to practice the double win. If I help you win, then I win. Winners profit from the past and guard their memories there. They set their goals just out of reach—not out of sight—to pull them where they want to go. They live in the only moment of time over which you and I have any control—the now.

You are a winner when the people you meet can say to you with honesty, "I like myself best when I'm with you."

Workbook for Day Twenty-five

ASSIGNMENT ONE: TEN POINTS OF POSITIVE MENTAL ATTITUDE

The following questions will help you to formulate thoughts for an effective life adjustment:

1. Check your personality temperature. Happiness is a byproduct, a result, of effective life adjustment. If you're not happy, what could you do to make your life more fun?
2. Do you have a zest for living? Can you be the developer of excitement and enthusiasm?
3. Are you socially adjusted? Do you like being and sharing with others?

4. Do you have balance and unity? Balance is needed when you find yourself wrapping your life around one thing or one person. Unity is doing something or not doing something and then refusing to worry about it.
5. Can you live with each problem in your life as it arises? Do you worry about the future or the past? Of all the things you worried about last year, how many of them came true?
6. Do you have insight into your own conduct? Insight means you know the real underlying reasons for what you do.
7. Do you have a confidential relationship with some other person?
8. Do you have a sense of the ridiculous—of what the world does to you? Can you laugh at yourself? If you look to see who laughs and who doesn't, you need to work in this area of your mental attitude.
9. Are you engaged in satisfying work?
10. Do you know how to worry effectively? Overcome your worries by going to the proper people for help.

A Day in the Life
JEAN

Thursday, 1 P.M. My sister arrived right before lunch and we ate together. People came over and commented on how much we look like each other, and for once that didn't irritate me, or her either apparently. She is scared and so am I.

Blanche asked us what we wanted to do, and we both were adamant about not involving our parents. We just don't think we would be believed. Blanche told us we needed to confront Uncle Joe because he is actively abusing a child, and Patti is probably not the only one. She says he has an illness over which he seems to exercise no control, and the only way his behavior can be checked is by breaking through the secrecy. Suddenly I started getting so angry! How dare this man have so much power in our family! I said I didn't care who knew, let them all suffer! Janet talked me out of it. She said that as Patti's mother, she was ready to call our uncle and confront him on the phone. She didn't want to put it to paper and was afraid to confront him in person.

Blanche said, "Do you have his telephone number?"

"You mean, now?" Janet said.

"I'll do it if you won't," I said.

Janet got very quiet. "No, this is my job."

Uncle Joe has never really held down a job. He dabbles in real estate and the stock market and has a home office, and he lives alone. Janet said, "I'll call him now." I asked her if she wanted me to be on an extension in case he got nasty. Janet said, "Yes, but we'll have to tell him. It wouldn't be fair otherwise." She's amazing. Always so concerned about things being fair! I went into the next room and left the door open so I could see Janet and she could see me. As she was waiting for the phone to ring, she said, "Oh, please, God, let him not be at home!" but before she got the final word out, he answered—that charming, oily voice of his.

"I've got something to say to you," Janet said in this businesslike way. "And Jeannie is on the line, too."

"That's right," I said, maybe too belligerently.

"What are you two up to now?" Uncle Joe said amiably. "What can I do for you?"

"You can keep your hands off my daughter for one thing," said Janet. Her voice was cool but shaking. There was a long pause on the other end of the line. "Did you think Jeannie and I didn't remember what you did to us when we were little? Did you think my daughter would be too afraid to tell me about what you did to her when we were home for Dad's illness? What gives you the right to sexually abuse little girls, Uncle Joe?"

"You're lying," he said, marvelously cool and collected. "You are both very, very sick. Who else have you lied to? I'll sue you for everything you're worth."

"I could sue *you* for what you've done," said Janet, "but I wouldn't put my child through that. But let me tell you something, if you ever lay a hand on her, or even look at her funny, I guarantee you, I will."

There was another long pause. I could hear his heavy breathing. Finally he said, "Have you told this to your mother and father?"

"Should we?" I said. "Why shouldn't they know? Why shouldn't everyone know so they can protect themselves?"

"No, we haven't," said Janet. "We're trying to keep the damage you've done to a minimum. Not even my husband knows, because if he did, he'd probably kill you. I want to hang up now."

I came into Blanche's room and the three of us held each other. Janet was sobbing. Blanche and I told her how terrific she was. "I lost my cool, but you didn't," I said. "You're wonderful."

That night I got a pass and we went to a silly movie, laughed our heads off, and then spent the night together in Janet's motel room. It was like a slumber party. We talked until nearly dawn, about everything and nothing. I have never felt so close to anyone. When she left, I cried so hard. We're bonded now. It's tragic it took an event like that to make it happen, but it proves to me the adage that there's something good even in the worst of things.

Or like this woman who qualified at an AA meeting who talked about incest. We can take what happened to us and put it into an ability to understand what it means to be oppressed, to know what it does to the victim, the twisted logic, the denial. She was working with the homeless she said, and she was grateful she was an incest survivor. It gave her a frame of reference for their suffering.

Day Twenty-six

STEP STUDY: STEPS FOUR THROUGH TWELVE

The Twelve Steps are a way of life and require action. They are not read so much as worked. The Step Study in this book is only a basic introduction to them, for they become more meaningful as you progress in recovery. Some people spend years working Step One. Others come into the program ready to work Step Twelve! There are no deadlines to meet. Everyone proceeds at the pace they feel they are ready for, although many people in the program use one step a year as a guideline.

The following is a synopsis of Steps Four to Twelve,

as an introduction, and to prepare you for what lies ahead. The beauty of the Twelve Steps is that they focus on you. They are concerned only with your own growth, for the sole purpose of making you "happy, joyous, and free." They are not dogma, only the most practical of applications of basic human principles to one's daily life.

By the time people have worked through Step Three, they have made a commitment to the program. They have acknowledged their powerlessness, that their lives have become unmanageable, that there is a power greater than themselves that they have tapped into and a need to relinquish their wills to this higher power. Until the results of surrender are experienced, when help does arrive as promised, through other people, and begins to work, restoring sanity to your life, the steps beyond the third will seem insurmountable. But power comes from tapping into this great resource that is available to all of us willing to surrender our wills, and it gives us an entirely new outlook on life. Suddenly, it *is* possible to change, and the energy required for it is there, in abundance. So read these steps with the realization that there is outside help in doing them. Otherwise you will feel too much is required. And don't *think* too much about them. Action is the key to this program, one day at a time. Miracles are common, but they do not just happen.

STEP FOUR

"Made a searching and fearless moral inventory of ourselves."

People recoil from this step. Suddenly they are hit with the realization that this program is going to require them to change, and they don't think they're ready. But without change, there is nothing. Pain isn't about change, it's about resisting change. The catharsis of the first three steps—when one experiences the great relief and joy of discovering there is help in the universe and that life's problems need not be dealt with in isolation—is not enough for recovery. Change begins within, with a strong searchlight beamed inward.

Inventory is not a critical evaluation. It is an assessment. It examines assets, finds out what there is enough of, too much of, and what is lacking in order to conduct business. A moral inventory is an examination of needs. When you are ready to take the Fourth Step, you will list your assets first and then take a look at your character defects, the things about you that cause negative consequences, and be ready to acknowledge them fully.

STEP FIVE

"Admitted to God, to ourselves, and to another human being the exact nature of our wrongs."

Step Five is a catharsis. It does not result in an overnight change, but it does bring the relief of having no more secrets to bear alone. In the process of accepting ourselves, with all our defects, our acceptance of others grows. We no longer expect perfection of anyone, especially ourselves.

STEP SIX

"Were entirely ready to have God remove all these defects of character."

This step is not as simple as it seems. We are secretly fond of many of our character defects and don't really want to give them up. The power God has to remove these defects is experienced at the point of surrender, when the insane craving for a mood-altering substance is lifted out. The miracle of that prepares us, although the removal of our character defects is more gradual and ongoing than the lifting of our craving for food.

STEP SEVEN

"Humbly asked Him to remove our shortcomings."

Humility is always difficult. To most people it equates to weakness, but it is nothing more than a desire to seek and do God's will, and our behavior will gradually and remarkably change.

STEP EIGHT

"Made a list of all persons we had harmed, and became willing to make amends to them all."

The person at the top of our lists should be ourselves, and learning to make amends to ourselves first will help us make amends to the others we have harmed, out of fear, resentment, sex, and pride. The inventory of Step Eight is even more difficult than that of Step Four, because it forces us to confront our deeds, and the pain we have caused, something we have probably worked hard to deny. The humility required of us in the previous step prepares us.

STEP NINE

"Made direct amends to such people wherever possible, except when to do so would injure them and others."

Sometimes making amends is easy. A child is listened to, a spouse is treated with respect, a debt is paid. Apologies are often in order, but amends are about action more than words. Behavior change means more than the most eloquent plea for forgiveness. In certain situations direct amends are not possible. The person harmed may have died. Someone who loved you may be in a new relationship, and hearing from you would reopen rather than heal a wound. Or a spouse might be greatly harmed to hear about your extramarital adventures. Each amend must be carefully evaluated, but when it is appropriate, screwing up one's courage and being forthright without getting excessively remorseful is the way to do it.

STEP TEN

"Continue to take personal inventory and when we were wrong promptly admitted it."

One of the characteristics of people who have been in a 12-step program for a long time is their willingness to admit they are wrong. It is such a rare thing in this world that they stand out as special. Admitting it promptly is possible if a daily inventory is taken, for carrying around the knowledge of a wrong committed against someone is poisonous, and it must be discharged. It's a lot easier to be ignorant of the wrongs we do, for awareness of them carries the responsibility of action. The benefit of acting in an esteemable way is worth the humility required by this step. We can be glad we are who we are, because we live honestly. We have nothing to hide, and nothing to be ashamed of, even our imperfections, for we readily admit them.

STEP ELEVEN

"Sought through prayer and meditation to improve our conscious contact with God as we understood Him, praying only for knowledge of His will for us and the power to carry that out."

Life becomes remarkably simple by the Eleventh Step. We don't need to make agonizing decisions about what we should do or not do, what course in life to take, whether we are doing the right thing or should be doing something else. All we need to do is pray for the knowledge of God's will for us (and that will always works in our favor) and the power to carry it out. After receiving that knowledge, and feeling that power, we are readily convinced that this is the way to live. It is in no way abrogating responsibility. It is seeing ourselves as connected to universal principles, being on the giving as well as the receiving end of a system of mutual benefit in which nothing is ever lost except trouble and nothing ever gained except joy.

STEP TWELVE

"Having had a spiritual awakening as the result of these steps, we tried to carry this message to [food addicts], and to practice these principles in all our affairs."

The spiritual awakening is experiencing the strength and serenity that comes from changing destructive behavior. When people are suddenly able to do things they couldn't do before, no matter how hard they tried; when they begin to feel life is worth living even though their circumstances may not have changed; when they realize there is more to life than what they thought—much more—they feel an urge to give to others what they have been so readily given themselves. The 12-step program works because people help each other stay in recovery. In fact, recovery is not possible without the Twelfth Step. You may have known people who are "dry alcoholics," who remain sober by the white-knuckle method, without AA. They are rarely happy people. Life is just as unhappy as when they were drinking, often worse, because now they have to deal with reality on an hourly basis. The Twelfth Step describes the difference—without a spiritual awakening and the willingness to help others, there is no recovery.

The Twelfth Step does not mean you stand on the corner and proselytize. This is an anonymous program, and it works because it is one of attraction, not promotion. The new person you are will inspire others, not what you tell them. But if there is someone you know who is gaining more and more weight, who looks miserable and acts helpless, don't wait for that person to approach you. Remember the isolation you felt before you sought help. Engage her in conversation. She may open up about her problem, or you might tell her about yours. If she is ready to be helped, you will know. If she rejects help, don't feel you have failed. You have planted a seed.

Practicing the Twelfth Step is a pure form of loving, for it asks nothing in return. Nevertheless, those returns are without measure—in a maturity of outlook, and a profound happiness, a circle of deep friends, and a purpose for being alive.

Workbook for Day Twenty-six

ASSIGNMENT ONE

Writing a Plan for Living: What is your attitude toward change and growth, having come this far? Are you committed to making some changes? Do you feel your reactions to life have changed from being introduced to the Twelve Steps, and do you know how these changes came about? To help you with these important questions, I encourage you to make some initial preparations. Try listing some of your defects, the attitudes and behaviors that are causing you the most trouble in your life. List some of your assets, too, and incorporate them into your plan for personal growth. What about your new program of spirituality?

Write this material down. Try to be as specific as possible in making your plan for living. *Then live it!*

A Day in the Life

ELAINE

Friday. My family left last night, but my daughter's coming back a week from Monday. She wants to enter treatment. I'm so thrilled! I know it's because she sees what this program has done for me. This morning we enacted codependency with Laura, a woman my age who takes on everyone's problems. The instructor, Marie, had Laura go around the circle and tell each person she would solve all their problems. We said things like, "Will you clean my house?" and "Will you find me a job?" and she kept saying, "Yes, I will," "Yes, I will." Then she leaned down in the center of the group and three people stood over her, pushing down on her shoulders until Laura asked them to please stop.

Marie said, "Do all these things people ask you to do get kind of heavy? Tell them what you want."

Laura said, "I'd like for you to begin to think for yourselves."

"But I like it the way it is," said one.

"Take care of me," said another.

"I'm not convinced," said a third.

Laura said, "It's hard for me to cut off my feelings of concern."

Marie said, "What do you need?"

Laura said, "To be whole, peace."

Marie said, "Start small," and Laura shouted, "I want them to get off my back!"

We all applaud. Then Marie said, "Now I want you to ask for help getting up."

"I've never done that before," said Laura. Marie asked her what's happening to her, in her gut. Laura said she's in pain. "I'm afraid I'm asking too much of them to help me up."

Marie said, "I hear you saying they're not capable. When you say you're asking too much, you're deciding for the other person that they're not capable of deciding for themselves. Take care of yourself and allow others to be who they are."

I really related to this dramatization. When we act things out, they become so clear. Even though we laugh, we're empathizing behind our smiles. I ask Marie why psychodrama is so powerful, and she says, "When you're in group therapy, you're yourself with all your defenses, but when you play a role, you're without them. Psychodrama cuts past those defenses straight to the emotions."

3 P.M. My last class with Ken. He talks about recovery. Warns us that people will expect our old behavior, and we've got to expect them to expect it until we show them otherwise. He says, "If they guilt-trip you as a reaction to your setting boundaries with them, use the Columbo Technique of Strategic Incompetence." Here's what that means: Say you get a real guilt-inducing message on your answering machine from someone who's upset you haven't called. Never call them back and say, "I'm sorry I haven't called." Instead of apologizing, say, "Hey, thanks for calling. I'm glad to know you can call if I don't call you and you won't just sit around and feel bad about it." Act happy, tell them they're competent. Use your own motivation, not the motivation of the guilt trip. Don't be so understanding. Be less responsible. That's the Columbo Technique of Strategic Incompetence.

On the bus to OA tonight I think back to the first trip, when I felt so isolated and uncomfortable. Why do I love these people so much? Maybe it's because we're vulnerable with each other. We try to be honest. We've cried in front of each other like babies. There's nothing any of them could say that I wouldn't try to understand. I don't have to agree with them to do that, but I can listen for the meaning and make human contact. I can sit on this bus and just be, watching the world go by, all those neon fast-food-restaurant signs that will soon be tempting me, and I can turn to Tony sitting next to me and say what's on my mind without having to put on the old Elaine act, the one that made me so exhausted. I can look at him with my naked face and say what's in my heart, and if he interrupts me, I know I can say, "Hey, when you don't let me finish my thought, I get annoyed. I need you to hear me out." Life is so much easier it makes me laugh to think about it.

Day Twenty-seven
AFTERCARE

In the new direction you're traveling, your windshield needs to be much bigger than your rearview mirror. What has happened to you is worth a watchful glance now and then, just to make sure it's not tailgating you in the present, but what lies right ahead—today—is your major concern.

What are your chances for staying in recovery? Better than with some diseases, worse than with others: The general statistics are that after treatment for addiction, one-third continue to struggle, going in and out of recovery, one-third go straight into recovery and stay there, and one-third relapse. The statistics for my program are better than the national average. By the number of letters I get from former patients, reporting in glowing terms of their permanent changes, I *know* what we're doing at Janet Greeson's "A Place For Us." I also know a well-worked-out program of aftercare can make all the difference.

You will be playing a new game in recovery, with new players. Baseball is the metaphor of the 12-step program for me. You're congratulated when you hit a home run, encouraged by your teammates. It's a gentle game, it moves at a slow pace with polite and elaborate protocol, and it doesn't hurt. Football is the game we played when we were active in our addictions, and it hurt. For a while—for the next ninety days—you're going to stay away from football fields and football players. You'll tell people you've learned to play a new game. You need to make your recovery the number-one priority in your life, because, believe me, **whatever you put before it, you will lose.** It's hard for people who are accustomed to putting everyone else's needs first to make themselves the number-one priority, but helping yourself first will make you much better at helping others later.

At our aftercare sessions at Janet Greeson's "A Place For Us," we form a circle and each person says, "I place my hand in yours, so we can do the things together I cannot do alone," until everyone in the circle is holding hands. You can't recover alone. For the next ninety days, you need a meeting every day. You need to call your sponsor every day. You need to take care of yourself and keep doing all the good things you're doing like regular exercise. If you take good care of yourself, the other things in your life will get taken care of, too, without the usual struggle. You will need to let go of relationships with people who don't respect you. You will need to keep the sickness of self-destructive and negative thoughts from creeping back into your mind. You will need to play the game of life with gentle people who abide by the rules that honor recovery.

At 12-step meetings, seek out the winners—the ones with long recovery who show enthusiasm and warmth—and follow them around. Avoid those who project negativity. They are an energy drain you can ill afford right now. This is no time to go around saving others, even if it does feel good to take the focus off yourself and put it onto someone who needs help even more than you.

You also need a specific plan for your aftercare, with dates and times and places. Fill out the forms in the aftercare worksheets in today's workbook with the kind of determination you have learned you are capable of, but don't get too ambitious. Remember, addiction is about extremes, and your tendency will be to throw yourself into this next step, particularly because you feel so good and powerful. But that way leads to relapse. **"Easy does it."**

Workbook for Day Twenty-seven

ASSIGNMENT ONE: AFTERCARE WORKSHEET

Draw a vertical line down the middle of a sheet of paper. On the right side write the word *Plan* and on the left the word *Goal;* on the goal side you will describe what you want to accomplish, on the plan side, how you are going to achieve your goals. Make these plans as specific as possible, with dates, times, and locations, so you don't get bogged down keeping an impossible schedule later.

Your first goal concerns food and other mood-altering substances. If your goal is to remain abstinent, your plan will specify how you will do so: by attending at least four meetings a week, for example, getting a sponsor, planning your meals or working the twelve steps. Other items to chart are:

—Family and friends
—Recreation and physical conditioning
—Occupation and education
—Spirituality
—Other

Go over this aftercare plan with someone in the fellowship, preferably your sponsor.

ASSIGNMENT TWO: SELF-EVALUATION

1. List three positive achievements that you feel you have accomplished in these twenty-eight days, physical as well as mental.
2. List three defense mechanisms that you can now recognize in yourself and some recent examples when using them affected you adversely.
3. List three new behavior patterns you are practicing to substitute for these negative behaviors.

A Day in the Life

TONY

Saturday. My last day. Vickie's group went to the mall on their pass this afternoon and came home with bright yellow T-shirts they had imprinted with the logo "Vickie's Victors." They argued about whether it should be "Vickie's Victims," but then Leslie, who went with them, said, "Hey, she'd get upset to hear you think of yourselves as victims." So they're going to surprise her in group on

Monday. Elaine, Gloria, Sam, and I went to a movie, then hung around the mall. Gloria is a changed person. She's still a wild character, but the nastiness is gone. She's so happy to be going into a halfway house and has found out it's just a few blocks away from Sam, who's sort of adopted her.

5 P.M. Dr. Shanks talks to us, a real inspiring guy. He's an MD and an addictionologist, and he used to weigh six hundred pounds. He talked about addicts in society, how we do everything with a little insanity, and how many famous artists in history were addicts. He says we have been given a gift, of extra sensitivity: "I never met a stupid addict." Says we should be thankful for our addictions. "Alcohol and food saved my life. They kept me from committing suicide." When we're ready, those of us who are lucky enough to find this program can save our lives by helping each other stay abstinent, one day at a time.

9 P.M. My wife should be landing at the airport any minute. Then, a little holiday at Disney World before reentry. We've got a lot of talking to do, and a lot of getting close. I told her she can get twenty-six pounds closer to me now, and she said, "I bet I can get a lot closer than that, if you give me a chance." My bags are packed, and I've said my good-byes. I have phone numbers and addresses of these people who mean so much to me. When I need to read some affirmations, I'll just read what they wrote about me.

The twenty-six pounds I've shed are not as important as the other things I'm leaving behind, like a gallon of tears, a sealed drum of stinking thinking, and enough kilowatts of anger to light the whole city for an hour. Thank you, God.

Day Twenty-eight
RECOVERY

> There is a destiny that makes us brothers; none goes his way alone. All that we send into the lives of others comes back into our own.
>
> —Edwin Markham

I like to say that we do the surgery in treatment, but real recovery takes place in the recovery rooms of the 12-step program. Before treatment, food addicts can be seen as victims of their disease. After treatment, if they choose to remain in their addiction, they're no longer victims. They've just sold out. They know there's a way out of their addiction, and for whatever reason, they choose not to follow it. You have now relinquished the right to be a victim and are responsible for making a choice between whether you wish to recover or stay addicted.

I agree with you that it's not an easy choice. Recovery is not a sudden landing. It is a process, and no one ever gets recovered, only remains in recovery. For thousands of years, addicts just died of their addiction, but to me, one of the miracles of the twentieth century is the 12-step program, developed by addicts, for addicts and run by addicts, for the sole purpose of helping them stay in the state of recovery. The reason it has flourished so phenomenally is simple: It works!

One of the common complaints of the nonaddicted is that when people join a 12-step program, they stop being addicted to a substance to become addicted to the group. There is some truth to this, for we addicts always do things in an extreme way. However, the need for meetings does not and should not remain at the high-intensity level that is necessary in early recovery. At a certain point, there is life beyond the rooms. During the detoxification phase, the body is still craving the substances it has been denied, the mind is not yet clear, and the unaccustomed state of reality is like a too-blinding light after years spent in a dark place. In this supersensitive phase, a meeting every day is essential—even more if the discomfort is great.

The first ninety days is a constant struggle, after which there is a period of triumph often called the "pink cloud" of early recovery. But the entire first year is a difficult time during which one priority is enough for anyone to handle—staying abstinent and going to meetings. Everything else should be put on the shelf and no major changes should be made, in jobs, relationships, or geographic moves. The first year is no time to fall in love, because the object of our affection is likely to be just that—an object—upon whom we channel all our thwarted obsessive behavior. Years of failed relationships in early sobriety has resulted in a 12-step rule—no relationships during the first year. Of course, everything is a recommendation in the fellowship. If newcomers follow their own rules, they won't be chastised, and when they then come tearful and devastated to a meeting after the relationship has ended badly, they will be comforted without anyone's admonishing them with an I-told-you-so.

People often ask, "How do I know when I'm in recovery?" If you have to ask, you're not. You can have abstinence without recovery. Abstinence is the opportunity for recovery. When all you're thinking and talking about is food, even if you're not abusing it, and when you're using food to hide who you really are, you're still in the addiction. People in recovery radiate it. They have no secrets to hide. Somebody's home and you're being invited in. They're willing to share what they've got. When you reach that state, you'll know it and so will others.

Another problem that's important to deal with in recovery is rigid thinking. One of the things people in early sobriety ask me the most is, "Do you mean I can't have a piece of cake or a cookie or a fudge brownie for the rest of my life?" I believe that's dangerous thinking. First of all, this is a day-at-a-time program. Secondly, it is this kind of extreme thinking that gets addicts in trouble. People should definitely remain abstinent from all mood-altering foods for a year, but after that, they have enough recovery under their belt to stop thinking in "never again" terms.

To avoid the rigid thinking that characterizes addiction, look for patterns. Take the seasons. They ebb and flow in a fixed way, but no one can predict exactly when summer's going to come. A basic to recovery is to set up a new pattern for a lifestyle you can live with, things you want to change, and to look at it as a natural force in the evolution of life instead of within the narrower scope of following a diet. We, too, ebb and flow like the seasons. Our moods change from day to day, but we are part of a pattern that has a purpose and a direction. It's not that summer won't come, it just comes in its own time and its own way. If we focus on the patterns, a healthy lifestyle and a healthy way of eating, instead of focusing on exactitudes and the rigidity of perfection, we can make life a lot more pleasant for ourselves.

Between three and five years into recovery, people begin to take on larger issues. Many go into therapy to deal with them. They can also expand their identity. The phrase "you are what you eat" is so limiting! You may carry the results of what you eat, but you are much more than that. Be sure you leave this treatment phase with a burning desire to find out who you really are. In the beginning it's important to identify ourselves as food addicts, but we need to go beyond seeing ourselves as people with an addiction to who else we are—sensitive, caring people with imagination, dreams, hopes, and thoughts, with something valuable to offer society because we have no illusions about ourselves.

It's not enough to follow the program. You have to learn to think and act responsibly. Otherwise people are just transferring their dependency from one authority to another authority and never learning to think for themselves and deal with unstructured time. There are people who use the program to avoid what's going on at home. To me that's not recovery.

Recovery is about style. It's about developing a style of living until it works. It's about not being afraid to tell people who you are because *you* know who you are and don't care if others like you because *you* like you. Recovery is about having a love affair with yourself so you can have one with life. It's about being happy, joyous, and free.

I wish you great joy and success in yours as I have in mine. If I can do it, you can do it, but none of us can do it alone.

Workbook for Day Twenty-eight

ASSIGNMENT ONE: MIRROR AFFIRMATION

Begin and end each day for the next ninety days by looking at yourself in the mirror and saying:

I love you.
You are brave.
You are full of courage and power.
You are one of the lucky ones.
You are willing to change.
I love you.
I am good to myself.
I care about me.
I want the best for me.
I want to be the magnificent person I am today.
I am full of love for myself and others.
There is more than enough for all.

ASSIGNMENT TWO: VISUALIZATION: MIRROR IN YOUR MIND

This visualization works best if you do it with your buddy, one of you reading while the other goes through the visualization, then reversing roles.

Prepare for deep meditation in the way you have been practicing for the past twenty-eight days. In your mind, approach a three-way mirror, wearing a favorite outfit, either in your current wardrobe or from your past. Stand in front of it in bright light and look yourself in the eyes. Smile and say hello. Be glad to make your acquaintance. With love in your heart, begin scanning your body as if you were really seeing yourself anew, for the first time—as if you had just met a delightful stranger.

Decide you want to get to know this stranger better. Study him or her: What does body language reveal? What kind of expression does the face wear the most often? What can you tell about this person by the clothing?

Admire this person: the way the hair falls, the lines of the leg and hip, the curve of the chest and shoulders. What a magnificent work of art you are! What a thing of beauty. You are truly God's child, a creature six million years in the making, capable of thinking as well as feeling, of dreaming of the future as well as remembering the past, able to become much more than you are if you choose.

Return to your eyes. Approach the mirror and look deeply into them. Say the words "I love you just the way you are."

You can do it. You can learn to love your whole being, as you are. Just because you have a forty-inch waist rather than a thirty-inch waist doesn't make you an unsatisfactory person. What counts is that you are caring, loving, kind, and first and foremost, good to yourself. You don't have to be model perfect to be a good person, but you do have to love yourself, and to be appreciative of what God has given you.

A Day in the Life

JEAN

Sunday. I'm still thinking about what Terry, the woman who does aftercare with us, said about my future. She says I have a real gift for writing. She's a jazz singer, with Artie Shaw and people like that. For a while, after she stopped drinking, she insisted she couldn't sing. Then one day her sponsor made her get up at a small club and just do it, just start singing, and she did, and sang better than ever. She's still singing in nightclubs. Terry tells me, "The point of attention determines the balance of power." As long as she was putting her attention on her inability to sing, she couldn't sing. As long as I put my attention on my past history of being unable to make it academically, I'll fail.

I've never thought about being a writer, but it's funny, I've been writing all my life, always scribbling down my thoughts. I remember something Ken said in class, that creative people often have an imposter syndrome because they have places they want to get to and they're not sure if they're there yet because it's a new place. New ideas, flying free, wild, and lonely, so the creative person says, "Could it be? Is this me?" Yeah, there's no checks, no cultural references. Where I am is new. It's exhilarating and confusing. Like when I performed the part of the little kid in the psychodrama "I'll Love You Forever" with Elaine as the mother. It was about how a little girl grows up, and no matter how she acts up, the mother rocks her at night and sings, "I'll love you forever, I'll like you for always, as long as you're living, my baby you'll be." Then, when the mother gets old, sick, and too weak to sing, the roles are reversed and the daughter rocks her as the chorus sings. By the end of the psychodrama, everybody was in rampant tears, people sobbing and wailing. I was close to tears, too, but I had so much fun acting. I really felt as if I were two, nine, a teenager, and a young woman. People said, "You were great." Their eyes were shining at me for what I did, said, am, but I don't remember what I did because I didn't plan it, control it, or own it. I am a vehicle for it. I told Ken this and he said, "Some people call it freedom." This place has done so much for my confidence. And I don't need alcohol to create, don't need any kind of drug. I'm high on this place.

8:30 P.M. Change. Something of people's auras hangs about their beds when they leave. I can see and feel mine, a cocoon of energy and a live moving spot, like a warm current in the ocean. Where Jill was is still Jill's aura, though there's a new, unsuspecting, scared woman here, like I was. I see a golden light by what was Debbie's door and feel pulled by her gulfstream into her room, expecting to enter the halo around Miriam's bed and be accepted and loved. They have been home a week and it's still their room to me. Miriam's carpet is cool and inviting, and I still feel her sensual electricity, her hot brooding. I still hear her deep laugh.

Now I sit in the capsule of light around my bed. I'm taking the blankets off, folding them, stripping the sheets. Maybe tomorrow, maybe tonight, someone new will occupy this bed, someone scared who knows nothing of me, and the process goes on. I take most of my love home inside of me, but I leave shadows of golden crystals under the bed, on a chair, in the air. This place has touched me and my life will never be the same. A place of healing is indelible, and the healing person is a messenger of love, a living legend of experience, strength, and hope. With sun on my wings I can fly.

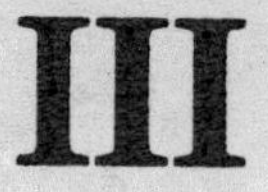

Recovering One Day at a Time

8

One Year Later, One Day at a Time

The addictive impulse is powerful; two out of three people who complete treatment relapse. The desire to abstain from use is the only requirement for membership in a 12-step fellowship. Relapse is losing that desire, but it can be rekindled at any time. Remember, abstinence is only the opportunity for recovery. The first human impulse is toward happiness, and addicts react to that impulse with typical intensity. As one person put it, "Serenity is the greatest high I've ever known."

Tony represents the one-third who leave a treatment center and go straight into recovery. He was a likely candidate with his respect for results, his love of simple cause-and-effect logic, the encouraging feedback he kept getting as he shed his weight, and his new relationship with his wife. Tony's willingness to be vulnerable and to let go of his need for control attracted him to her more than ever, and she told him she now felt really close to him, "like buddies." Because he could tell her what he needed, she relinquished her victim role as cancer patient in remission and became a true helpmate. Today they describe themselves as deeply in love.

Tony was also fortunate to have a support group all but waiting for him at the airport, for an immediate plunge back into relapse is common. His secretary gave him a list of Overeaters Anonymous groups, and he finally found one he liked that meets at noon near his office. He rejected some groups for being "too judgmental." "Food addicts wear their disease, unlike drinkers and pill poppers," he explained. "You have to be careful in OA not to be in a group where a lot of people judge others by what they look like. People don't do that in the AA groups I've been to, and they shouldn't do it in OA either. It's bad enough the world judges us for what we look like. My home group is very loving and accepting." Tony eventually modified his food plan "to feel more in control of it," but was consistent about avoiding white carbohydrates. He lost one hundred pounds his first year and is now a sponsor, a mainstay of his group.

Because Tony has made peace with his brother, who is now chief operating officer of the family company, he no longer takes on the entire responsibility for the business. He has more time to spend with his family and has taught his son how to flycast. Today Tony calls himself a happy man, "a miracle."

Elaine represents the one-third who go in and out of recovery before they finally make it. After two months, she binged on the way home from work, pulling into a 7-Eleven store after a particularly grueling day in which she had been criticized by her boss. She recalls, "Before I even started the car, I tore into that box of cookies and ate every one, then tossed the package into a garbage can in the parking lot." She then went off her food plan for a few days and stopped making phone calls to her sponsor. Then she stopped going to meetings. After two weeks she was so miserable feeling the pounds creep back around her stomach and thighs that she went to a meeting to share what was happening to her. She started out with the words "You see, I'm not perfect," and found she immediately had everyone's sympathy in the room.

A year later, Elaine is seventy-five pounds thinner, is working out at a local gym, and is able to communicate her real self to her son and daughter, who respond in kind. She has regular "dates" with each of them during which they share deep thoughts, and she is passionately in love for the first time in her life with her husband of thirty years.

Jean is currently in relapse. She lacked many of the stabilizing factors present in the situations of Tony and Elaine, particularly a loving spouse. At first, things went well for Jean. Instead of going to her family for more money, she got a job as a model-receptionist at a fashion designer's showroom, and she went to night school at the local college to earn a degree in journalism. She worked with incredible energy, putting all her obsessive-compulsive addictive behavior into her studies. Losing weight was easy when she put in sixteen-hour days. She ate a lot, didn't gain weight, and maintained her abstinence from refined carbohydrates, drugs, and alcohol. She began to feel invincible and even questioned whether she was really an addict after all.

It was family relationships that led to Jean's relapse. Several months after treatment she received a telephone call from her mother, who expressed great shock over the terrible rumors Jean had been spreading about Uncle Joe, who had never been anything but a darling man and a perfect gentleman. She told Jean, "The only explanation I can think of is that your drug-taking has caused you to lose your mind." Until Jean recanted and apologized to her uncle, she could never come home again.

After the phone call Jean took a nap and slept until late that evening, when she heard from one of her drugging friends. By midnight she was somewhat high on two lines of cocaine. Her reaction to the drug was complex. As Smitty had warned, the program had screwed up her drug-taking forever. The feeling was anxious more than euphoric, and her stomach contracted in disappointment that she should have so blithely thrown away four months' clean for a few minutes in an altered state, particularly when that turned out to be the state of despair. But at least her drugging friends were happy. She had returned to the fold, assuaging their own worries.

The cost of her nearly 120 days of sobriety was too great to lose on just a one-night bender. Jean relapsed with a vengeance. Vodka tonics followed, the imported beers she had missed so much, and lots of champagne at weddings, getting publicly tipsy and knowing that people were remarking she was off the wagon again. One day she resumed buying her own drugs, tired of hanging around users and hoping for a freebee. She experimented and found speed and alcohol elevated her mood better than cocaine and were cheaper.

Along with the bender went bags of Fritos, pints of Ben and Jerry's crushed Heath Bar ice cream, a resumption of caffeinated-coffee drinking—whole pots of it, like before—and in public, double espresso. Jean even resumed cigarette smoking after ten years. She wrote in the journal she still kept, "It seems all my old desires came roaring out of nowhere, overwhelming me."

One night Jean dreamed of herself as a little girl running down a road, fully alive. The next morning, she called the treatment center. Her heart began racing as soon as she heard Blanche's cheerful voice at the other end of the line.

"I've been thinking about you. How're you doing?"

"I relapsed," said Jean, and poured out the story of her mother and the phone call.

"Her response shows the power of the secret," Blanche said. "She's putting on you the guilt and shame her brother should be feeling. Think how angry you must be!"

Jean returned to the hospital for another four weeks of treatment. Her sister and mother came down for family therapy, and after many bitter hours during which her mother remained steadfast in her loyalty to her brother, she admitted she was also a victim of his sexual abuse, and she poured out her guilt over pretending it had never happened to her daughters. They became deeply bonded over the issue that had previously driven them apart, and

Jean left therapy hopeful she would be able to stay in recovery.

But she did not. One year later, she has relapsed four times, the last time dropping out of sight. The sexually abused must struggle against great odds to get out of the prison of their past, and they often fail many times before they succeed. But as Jean says, "We have guardian angels. You know that song 'God bless the child that's got its own'? It's true." Although Jean represents the one-third who do not recover from their addiction, she is still free to choose to surrender.

When Jean first relapsed, she heard the voice of Ken saying over and over, "Before treatment you were a victim. Afterward you just sold out." There is a new weight of responsibility to bear in relapse. Breaking the bonds made with the newly emerging self feels like the ultimate betrayal, a wounding of this brave and trusting "real you" who has been coaxed forth with such difficulty. The recriminations that rain down as fallout of these feelings of betrayal add to the anguish of relapse.

People in this state have the best chance of getting back into recovery if they stay connected with their sponsor, even if they are "active." Some people in the fellowship will shun them, for relapse is threatening to those who are insecure about their own sobriety. This leads people in relapse to feel like lepers, as if their behavior were contagious. Remember, the program is made up of a lot of sick people trying to help each other, and a lot of them may not be up to the task. But some will be, particularly those with long sobriety who suffered frequent relapse in the beginning, the ones who say, "My weakness became my strength." If people in relapse will come to meetings and ask for help, the people they need to find the most will find them.

Relapse is often described as purgatory, but it's not. It's insanity, and the only way out is with a pull from above. I don't believe you can get back into recovery without a spiritual connection. People in relapse think God has turned his back on them. The truth is, they have turned their back on God, and all they have to do is turn around again and ask for help.

9

Janet's Story

". . . What is Real?" asked the Rabbit one day.

"Real isn't how you are made," said the Skin Horse. "It's a thing that happens to you."

"Does it hurt?" asked the Rabbit.

"Sometimes," said the Skin Horse, for he was always truthful.

"Does it happen all at once?"

"You become real. It takes a long time. But once you are Real you can't become unreal again. It lasts for always . . ."

From *The Velveteen Rabbit*
by Margery Williams.

I was born in the Red Hook section of Brooklyn, in a working-class Irish neighborhood, as World War Two was coming to a close. My father was in the Army, and my mother was my universe. I was her first child. My earliest memory dates from age four when my life, which had been tranquil up to that point, took an alarming turn. My mother went to the hospital to give birth to my brother, and instead of the few days of life without her I had been prepared to endure, I was told she was sick and would be gone for ten days.

I was taken to my paternal grandmother's house in Queens, which to a child from Red Hook was like going to a foreign country. With her French-German accent, even my grandmother seemed foreign to me. Although she had a glorious garden with every kind of flower imaginable, and a fine house surrounded by soft green grass, my grandmother was cold and rigid. She was of the opinion that her son had married beneath him, and I always had the feeling there was something different about me that couldn't be discussed. Also, having lived by herself for many years, she was not at all comfortable around children, even one she might have approved of more than me.

I had to sleep with her. She had a habit of slathering her wrinkles with Noxema right before going to bed, and I lay every night feeling as if I were being gassed by the fumes. To this day I can't bear the smell of Noxema.

Then, when the ten days had finally passed, my grandmother told me my mother was home from the hospital but still too sick to care for me, and an eternity slowly passed while she did nothing but listen to the radio. The favorite thing for my mom and me to do was go to the movies. Finally I got my grandmother to take me to one, where I caused a ruckus, hoping she would think I was so horrible she would take me back to my mother.

My plan didn't work. As the days passed, I grew increasingly fearful that I would never see my mother again. Finally, after three interminable weeks, I was so desperate I decided to end my life. I found a rope and tied one end to the top of the cellar door, the other around my neck, and jumped. My grandmother found me and was so upset she hit me. After that she never let me out of her sight. Although I had rope burns on my neck, she never told anyone what had happened and neither did I. It became a secret.

Although I didn't want to be separated from my mother, she was difficult to be attached to, and more so after my brother came along and I had to share her attention. I can still see her, very obese then and usually alone, lying in bed reading romance magazines. I remember feeling as though if I took care of myself, it would be a help to her. My mother never knew the luxury of childhood, for she had nine brothers and one sister and pretty much raised the boys. In spite of her being surrounded by people all the time, I saw her as an isolated, lonely woman.

Although I always carried with me a fear that if something happened to my mother I would die, the message I received from her was clear: *You're a big girl now. You can take care of yourself.* We lived in a housing project, and every morning she would tell me, "Go out and play," but when I went downstairs, I couldn't find any children there because it was too early. One of the benchmarks of my life is standing in the courtyard looking up at hundreds of windows and feeling very alone.

But I could take care of myself. I was a big girl. When I went to kindergarten, my mother walked me to school the first day, a long walk through Coffey Park. After a few days she said, "You can go by yourself now. Get somebody to cross you," so I used to stand on the street corner and wait for some other kids to come with their mothers to get across the street.

We moved to South Brooklyn when I was in first grade, but I finished out the year in the school in Red Hook, taking a city bus to the old neighborhood for two months by myself. In the process I became a very independent child.

While my mother gave me the message that I could take care of myself, my father gave me another: *Be responsible, work hard, achieve great things.* He did all these things and had a good job working for the Transit Authority as a trainmaster. He was a big, strong man, outgoing and attractive to the women. I can see him at night in his chair, disappearing into one of the six or seven books he read every week. Although he was there, he was absent, and I yearned for contact with him. I thought I would win his love by being responsible, working hard, and achieving great things, but there was no real intimacy between us. I went to the movies once with him when I was nineteen. That's the only thing I can remember ever doing with him, just the two of us.

The thrill of my life, and the most intense source of love, was my maternal grandfather. I was crazy about him. He was brilliant, charming, and a roaring alcoholic. People loved him and took care of him. I actually remember wishing he was my father. I would say that if I ever wanted to be like anyone, I wanted to be like him. I don't ever recall my grandfather working, but I have many fond memories of him cooking meals, in which he took great pride. He loved to tell people how much I ate, and it was an easy way to get his approval. I even ate sardine sandwiches, which would repulse most kids, but I ate them for him.

He loved to take me to all those great Irish bars under the Myrtle Avenue el. I would stand on the bar, singing and dancing, a real little Shirley Temple, surrounded by laughing, approving men, getting money from them, and my grandfather getting drunk on the money and me on the attention. I couldn't get enough of that. On the way home he would always say, "Don't tell your mother where we've been," which made our trips to the bars all the more exciting.

There was another secret we shared that weighed much more heavily on my small mind, and that I knew without his saying a word should never be revealed. "Let's take a nap," he would say. I knew he was doing something wrong, but I loved him so much, and the conflict was intense. He was the only one in my world who seemed exciting to me, and because of our secrets I felt I was special. Without him I was nothing. I was only five or six years old, but I learned to live with the conflict.

The new neighborhood was more friendly and less crowded than the projects: two rows of brownstones with the focus on the street, which belonged to the kids. It was a safe place, and it rang with the noise and laughter of children in every kind of weather. On warm days and nights, grown-ups sat on stoops up and down the street and watched out for us. I was raised by an entire block of neighbors, most of them related to each other, forming a real clan right there in the middle of Brooklyn, and it was a great life.

Along with my Irish relatives and neighbors, there were a lot of Italians on the block, and they liked to cook pasta for me because I was such a hearty eater. One of my favorites was baked macaroni and cheese. Food was an expression of love that worked two ways: the pleasure I gave others because of the large amounts of food I was willing to consume for love, and the approval they gave me for eating it. Of course, I was obligated to eat it all and was glad I had an appetite that was up to the task, since that appetite was emotional, not out of true hunger.

In my family, eating and drinking to excess was a way of life. My mother, my grandmother, and my great-grandmother were all obese. When my great-grandmother died, they had to break a window and take her out like a piano because they couldn't get her through the door. While the women ate, the men drank. There was a lot of violence, a lot of chaos, and always a lot of food, which was highly valued by people who had experienced many long years of deprivation during the Depression and then the shortages of World War Two.

I was spirited, a leader, and excelled at everything I did. I channeled a lot of my energy into sports, where I learned to become a team player, and it was a great way to get the attention I craved. There was always part of me that was a maverick, and another part of me that wanted to lead people and be around them. I felt happiest when surrounded by people, but even then, racing to get my teammates out of the prison zone without getting tagged, with kids and babies and grown-ups all around, inside I always felt lonely and bad, a sense of shame I never understood. All I knew was, somehow I would never be enough.

I know today where those feelings came from. My mother and I were bonded in a way I didn't know then, by a man—her father and my grandfather—who sexually abused us. That was the origin of the shame, a mirror image, and the loneliness was bonding with a woman who had never completely bonded with anyone else. Today, having shared our secrets, we *are* bonded, by a love that goes much deeper than our mutual pain. Having been less than the perfect mother I wanted to be, I am now able to embrace her unconditionally. We work together, see each other nearly every day, and share a rich, full life.

But then I didn't understand. I only felt the shame and the loneliness and never believed I was enough.

When my father left for work, my mother would say, "Let's order a pizza." It was always the two of us, plus food. We ate well and often. A full meal would be followed two hours later by ordering out Chinese food. My mother was generous but she didn't share. If you wanted a slice, she would buy you a pizza, but she wouldn't give you any of hers. If you wanted one of her M&Ms, she would buy you your own bag, a big one. Food was too important to share.

Television became an important part of Brooklyn life in my growing-up years. Although my father was usually too busy reading, he watched *Kraft Playhouse Theater.* It was the only time the entire family watched television together. I still vividly recall the cheese commercials, the dishes floating magically before our eyes. I would buy the cheese for my mother and she would make the recipes. To this day I have a great affection for cheese. Maybe it connects me to that time and the presence of my father, his attention diverted from his usual solitary activity to focus with his family on those powerful commercials.

It's strange how many of my most vivid childhood memories are about feelings I had in connection with food. I wanted to be a part of something, connected, bonded. When I went to my maternal grandmother's house, I was always encouraged to raid her refrigerator, but she would tell me, "Save the pineapple juice for Uncle Eddie." Out of spite I would sneak into the kitchen and drink some straight from the can, trying to get away with as much as I could without being noticed. To this day I love pineapple juice and can never drink it without thinking about how I had to save it for Uncle Eddie, still wondering: How come I had to save it for him? Was pineapple juice too good for me?

I grew up tall, and because of my hyperactivity, I didn't really have a weight problem for many years. I was obsessed with sports, ballet, tap dancing, and never performed any of them in moderation. During summer vacations I played from ten o'clock in the morning until nine o'clock at night. I played basketball with the Police Athletic League and the YMCA and won all kinds of championships.

I excelled in school as well as in sports, although I never, ever studied. I started drinking around the age of twelve, and by my midteens was a real party girl. I loved the euphoria alcohol put me in. A new drink came out called the screwdriver. The first time I tried it, I had about twenty of them and blacked out. From that moment on I was a vodka baby.

I was skipped a grade in high school and graduated when I was fifteen. Instead of going to college, I wanted to join the Navy. Living close to the Brooklyn Navy Yard, sailors had always been a big part of my life, ever since my bar-hopping days with my grandfather, and I wanted to get a sailor. I didn't want to be an officer because I didn't think they had the fun that real sailors did, and I thought an education would lock me out of that. After graduation, working in the Greenwich Savings Bank until I was old enough to join the Navy, I lived the high life. Although I went out with hundreds of sailors in my teenage years, I never had sex with them. My mother had explained the facts of life to me at an early age and told me not to trust men. "They'll tell you they love you, but the only thing they're after is your cherry." I really believed it, not just because of my mother's warning, but because I saw that my sexually active girlfriends were always jumping from one man to the other without getting the respect I craved.

As soon as I turned eighteen, I went to the Navy recruiting office, where I was told I had to lose twenty pounds before they would take me. That was my first diet. It was simple: I didn't eat for ten days, danced a lot, and lost twelve pounds. When I went in for my physical, the recruiters were so impressed they figured I would lose the rest in boot camp and inducted me.

As soon as I was approved, I started eating until I reached 190 and had to get down to 170 to get into boot camp. In boot camp I was put in the Pudgy Platoon with all the people who had to take off weight. When the Pudgy Platoon was marched to chow, we went in the back of the line and got no bread, potatoes, or desserts, just meat and vegetables. I spent a great deal of my time in boot camp negotiating: "If you'll give me your bread and your dessert, I'll do your ironing." There was no way I was going to give up my food.

My job in the Navy was similar to what I had done at the bank because I was really bright when it came to math and accounting. I was in payroll. There was a lot of power in being in disbursing, close to the money. I traveled, to Norfolk, Newport, St. Albans, San Diego. At last I had left behind the reclusive life my mother lived, which I despised. It had always been inconceivable to me that she had never even been to see the Statue of Liberty.

At first everything was great. My life was so exciting—men, alcohol, parties, crazy times, feeling worldly. Everywhere I went I was popular and dated a lot, and because I wasn't the type to just jump in bed with anybody, I had a lot of sustained relationships. Nearly everyone drank a lot, and I certainly didn't believe I had a problem with alcohol, although the trouble I did get into almost always involved alcohol. When I'd be late or fall asleep and get restricted, losing my liberty pass, I'd climb into someone's trunk and get them to drive me out the gate.

After two intense years of the high life, I began to think my life was deteriorating. My drinking was now out of control and I had gained a hundred pounds. I started finding myself in uncomfortable situations with people I didn't want to be with, seedy people. I felt superior to them, that I was lowering my standards, and feared if I stayed in the Navy I would start sinking into a bottomless pit. One night, falling deeper and deeper into this state, I thought of my father and decided my problem was a lack of responsibility. If I was married and had children, I would have to act differently.

Driven by my father's message, I called up a man I had known all my life. He was in the Navy, of course, and seven years older than myself. Every time he had come home on leave when I was growing up, we went out together. He soon proposed. I accepted. I knew he loved me and it didn't matter if I loved him. After all, who else was going to marry me at 268 pounds?

I was twenty years old when I got married. My wedding gown was a size 48, and so heavy it bent the hanger. People told me I had a pretty face, and hearing that always made me feel awful, for it negated the rest of me. Shortly after the wedding, I got pregnant and my husband was deployed overseas. Suddenly I was alone for the first time, minus my customary social life, soon to be a mother, and without the faintest idea of how to really live. I felt as if I were dying. I had exchanged identities, giving up the party girl for the wife.

Worst of all, I was back in the old neighborhood. My husband's family lived across the street. Between my husband and me, we probably had fifty family members living on the same block, but I was not close to them the way I had been with the people I had been stationed with in the Navy. Like Alice in Wonderland grown too big for her house, I could not fit into that old life anymore. I had seen too much of the world. In spite of the close contact, there was no real intimacy, and I felt trapped.

I went through pregnancy and childbirth without my husband. He was gone for a year and a half. Old feelings of abandonment were tapped into and magnified a hundred times. My misery was so great, my addictions to food and alcohol began to take over my life. The responsibilities of marriage and motherhood had not rescued me, only made my need to alter my state of mind all the more urgent. The alcohol made me feel good, but when it made me feel bad, I used the food to feel good again. When I got sick from drinking too much, I ate to feel better, so no matter how I felt I was either eating or drinking to excess, and my weight mushroomed to 340 pounds. The bigger I got the more invisible I felt, for I had lost my identity under all that fat. I didn't feel I deserved to live and was slowly trying to kill myself.

When my husband finally returned, he got stationed at a Navy base in Lakehurst, New Jersey, and I went with him, thrilled to be out of my old Brooklyn neighborhood. Two years after the birth of Gene, I had another child, Jimmy. On the base I met a childhood friend with whom I used to run around in my party days. She was also stationed there with her husband. We got together and it was party time all over again.

I have a friend who says a social drinker is someone who every time someone says they want a drink, says, "So shall I." I was like that. I really believed that social drinking was drinking with people, telling myself I didn't have a problem because I never drank alone or in the morning. Also, I never drank at home unless I was having a party, telling myself only alcoholics drank at home.

Although I didn't want to stop drinking, I had a great desire to lose weight. I thought if I were thin, I could get my life back. I went to a doctor on Eastern Parkway in Brooklyn, who treated obesity with shots of pregnant women's urine and a diet of 300–500 calories a day, and lost a hundred pounds in four months. My seven-year marriage had been shaky for some time, and it ended with my weight loss. Shortly thereafter I met Charlie. Unlike my first husband, who was an alcoholic who didn't drink, Charlie was a Marine, an active alcoholic and lots of fun. I loved him and he was crazy about me. He was probably more like my grandfather than anyone I had ever known, not just in looks but in personality, too. I was in heaven, which for me was a place that was exciting, chaotic, and unpredictable.

My daughter, Rosemary, was born in 1970 and we moved to Florida. There Charlie and I had a classic alcoholic marriage. We brutalized each other. He was physically abusive when he was drunk, and I never knew what would upset him. He started combining alcohol with drugs and became even more unpredictable.

Meanwhile, I lost the same hundred pounds three times. I was always either on a starvation diet or putting the pounds back on that I had just lost, faster than I had lost them, plus a few extra. I went on the Stillman diet, I went to Elaine Powers. I went to TOPS, where I frequently took home the pig, given to the person who had lost the least amount of weight that week. I went to Weight Watchers. The instructor told us we had to take the skin off the chicken we ate and I made a face. She pointed a finger at me and said. "That's why you're fat." I was mortified and told myself. "I'll show that bitch." I lost weight for a little while, but for the wrong reasons.

I exercised like a fiend. I went to all kinds of diet doctors, and most of them gave me pills. Sometimes I'd go to three doctors at the same time and take all the pills, believing that whatever was going to work, if I took more of it, it would work better. One doctor I saw was morbidly obese. He handed me a prescription for pills and said, "These will work for you." I thought, How come they don't work for you then? but didn't say anything, afraid I wouldn't get the pills. I had to have that magic.

But there was no magic. Everything I tried failed. I had become a chronic dieter, either miserable on one or miserable because I wasn't on one. As soon as a diet set up the deprivation pattern, I was kicked into the internal void I had lived with all my life, that hole inside me that made me angry and full of despair. I am convinced that my reaction to that deprivation caused me to be heavier than I ever would have been had I not dieted at all.

When I was at my heaviest, my husband and I took a vacation to the Bahamas and boarded one of those small planes that take you from one island to another. I sat in the back as I did wherever I went, not wanting to be noticed. The plane taxied around the runway several times and then went back to the terminal. As my husband and I started wondering aloud whether there might be some mechanical difficulty with the plane, the stewardess approached us and asked me to move to the front of the plane and lean toward the middle. I was so heavy the plane was off balance and they couldn't get it off the ground!

I was mortified, and so was my husband. A normal person would probably have taken a vow at that moment never to binge again. Not me. The first thing I did when I got off the plane was eat. I had to numb out, and I continued to eat my way through the Bahamas because I kept worrying about how I was going to get back. The humiliation triggered the memory of other similar experiences, like the time I got stuck on a log flume ride in Coney Island because the machinery jammed. They made everyone get off except me and this nervous skinny guy. I couldn't get off and the ride continued. By the time I made the splash, it seemed as if a cast of thousands had gathered, hooting and clapping. I was dying inside then, too, and went straight to Nathan's and had popcorn, hot dogs, shrimp—anything I could get my hands on to numb those awful feelings.

After the Bahamas debacle, I went crazy with my eating. I would buy a loaf of Italian bread, make a hero, and eat the whole thing. Sometimes I would just chew my food and not swallow it. Then I discovered if I ate enough jelly doughnuts, I could bring them right back up again. I went to a clinic where I drank a solution and they pinched and pushed the fat out of you. I was nearly kneaded to death and didn't lose a pound. Whatever magical cure I heard for taking off weight, I tried it, making pilgrimages from place to place. I was going to have an intestinal bypass but decided not to because a friend of mine made an appointment first and told me the doctor had warned her there was a 10 percent chance she would die from the operation. I thought, with my luck I didn't dare risk the odds.

I read in the paper about a woman in Italy who glued her teeth together to lose weight. She lost a hundred pounds, plus her teeth. Then one day I was watching Phil Donahue interview a woman who had lost weight by having her mouth wired shut and drinking regular Pepsi. I was amazed at that, wondering why anyone would waste calories drinking regular soda. Still, I thought the idea was fascinating and decided it was my last resort.

I called a lot of dentists in Orlando. Most of them laughed at the idea and refused. Finally I found an oral surgeon who said he would do it for me. "Do you want to have your jaws wired tomorrow?" he asked. I told him I had to go on a vacation first. I went to New Orleans and Houston and put on another twenty-five pounds.

The procedure was excruciating. Sometimes I wonder whether the doctor didn't make it more painful than necessary as a deterrent. He put wires through my gums on the top and the bottom, attached them to a bar, then wired the two bars together. After three days I was banging my head against the wall, wanting something to hurt more than my mouth did. I took my son to Sea World, thinking that if I was around people I wouldn't cry. I cried anyway. Then the pain started to subside somewhat and I started suffering for other reasons. After three weeks of a liquid diet I was crazed. I started pulling at the wires, creating a little hole through which I could stuff food. It would take me hours to eat what I would normally consume in ten minutes.

When I went to the dentist to have my teeth cleaned, I watched him take the wires off in the mirror so I could figure out how to do it myself. It was difficult, because I had to reverse the process I saw in the mirror, but I managed to take them off, binge, and then wire them up again so nobody would know, then pray I wouldn't throw up from all the food I had been eating and choke to death. I knew what I was doing was insane, but I just had to have that food. I couldn't stand what was going on. My drinking increased as my food intake decreased, and I began to deteriorate physically. I ended up with alcoholic neuritis and could hardly walk.

Looking back, I see that period as my bottom. I wanted to die and couldn't, but I didn't want to live. My life was utterly out of control. In desperation I went to yet another overeaters' group, this time at the Orlando civic center. A friend of mine had told me about it, and I went with her and my mother. We went to the wrong location, and by the time we arrived the meeting had already begun. I sat in the back, taking up two chairs, in the vain hope I wouldn't be seen. It was January and cold but I was sweating and a nervous wreck. The speaker said to me, "You're late." I cringed and looked around for the diet. There wasn't one. That made me uncomfortable and intrigued at the same time.

The speaker told her story and then started talking about God. An atheist in the meeting started arguing with her, joined by an agnostic and a Jesus freak. I sat in the back on my two chairs, thinking, "What the hell's going on? Where's the diet?" I didn't even know what an agnostic was, and what did God have to do with losing weight? Then another woman, obviously from New York by her accent, spoke about how she had lost 112 pounds—not over and over like I did, but more or less permanently. I decided I didn't like her. She was too aggressive.

As soon as the meeting was over, I said to my mother and my friend, "Let's go eat." We went to a restaurant, stuffed ourselves, and laughed disparagingly at everybody at the meeting, the argument over religion, and the lack of a diet. I couldn't believe what I had witnessed, but I kept thinking about the woman from New York who said she had lost 112 pounds and not put them back on. That kept running through my mind, together with something someone had said about love. It hit home, as I had always connected food and love. And so I went back.

The next week the woman from New York started following me around. "Can I help you? Is there something I can do to help you?" she kept saying. I ignored her. She was the last person I wanted to be around, and I thought she was too pushy. That meeting the topic was feelings, and a lot of people were crying. I started to cry, too, and said to myself, What's happening to me? This is powerful, and when a list came around with people's names and phone numbers, I signed it.

The woman from New York called me every day. She asked me what I was going to eat that day and I wouldn't tell her, so she asked me what I had eaten. I started sharing that with her. She kept pursuing me in spite of my defiance and wouldn't give up on me. Beneath my front was a fearful woman who needed to have someone go after her. The addict in me didn't want to change, but the submerged healthy person in me desperately did, and during that struggle the woman called me every day.

The addict in me wanted magic, drama, chaos, and extremes, and not a slow process. Going to meetings and talking on the telephone every day was none of what my addict wanted, but there was someone else living inside me who desperately wanted to get better, and I kept going back.

The woman from New York saved my life. Except for that uncomfortable moment at my first meeting when I was accused of coming in late, no one in the group had judged me. I didn't have to look like Twiggy to be accepted by them. I didn't have to look like anybody. I was okay just the way I was.

In that atmosphere of acceptance, I started following instructions, willing to acknowledge the fact that my way obviously wasn't working. It wasn't education about food I needed. I knew what to eat and what not to eat. I needed a change in attitude, and I got that following the program, doing the assignments I was given, and going to meetings. I wanted to live instead of exist and knew I wouldn't be doing either for long if I didn't lose weight. There was something in the eyes of the people who went to the meetings that kept me coming back. They were real. I felt closer to some of them than others, but they were all real. They had all been through Death Valley and come out laughing.

I lost a hundred pounds that first year, and fifty pounds the next. I had experienced dramatic weight losses before, but this time it was different: I kept the weight off, month after month and year after year. Another thing was different: I was learning to like who I was, even when there was three hundred pounds of me, so when I came in contact with my slimmer self, I wasn't terrified of who that person was, as I had been before. It was still just me and I was okay. At a certain point, my intense craving inexplicably went away. I simply didn't need food to make me feel good anymore. I had learned how to do that by valuing and taking care of myself.

Instead of being addicted to food, I became addicted to meetings, and that was okay. After all, I'm an addict, and in the early years of my recovery I was compelled to do something in the extreme. I got extremely active. I became another pushy lady from New York who followed terrified newcomers around, asking, "Is there anything I can do to help you?"

My husband was not happy about my new self. In fact, he was threatened by it. The more weight I lost, the more insecure he became. When I was eating addictively, even though I was miserable, our relationship was comfortable in its familiarity. Because my eating was out of control, I was full of fear and felt powerless, completely dependent on my husband. He earned a good income as a career officer, and I hadn't worked for years. I hated having to count on someone else for financial survival and knew I had to prepare myself for being on my own. I desperately wanted to be responsible for my own life, and I knew education was my only ticket out. Charlie didn't want me to go to college but agreed to my attending motel-hotel school. When I told one of my instructors I was proud of the grades I got, he told me, "You don't belong here. This is nothing to you. You need to go to college."

One year into recovery from my food addiction, my perceptions of what I was capable of accomplishing changed and I gave up alcohol. That was too much for my husband to handle. He had often told me he would leave me if I got sober, and he made good on his threat. We had been living and raising three children on an income of $22,000 a year. That dropped to $5,000 a year once he left. I got very sober. I had a little money stashed away, plus a savings account for my children's education. That plus a job waitressing paid the bills.

As painful as that time was, my children and I were closer than ever. When my addictions were controlling me, I had been irritable a lot of the time and it was easy to take out my anger on them. Sometimes if they dropped a crumb on the floor, I would turn into a maniac. Gene told me he was grateful for my changes. When I was active in my addictions, he wouldn't bring any friends to the house because he never knew when I might go off on a tangent, and he was afraid to be around me most of the time. After I went into the fellowship he told me he'd rather be around me than anyone in the world. A lot of the anger had been an expression of my feelings of powerlessness, but flying into a rage had no place in my new perception of myself. Getting close to my children was one of the greatest gifts of my new life. My strength infused them, which in turn increased my own, and we all benefited from the changes I had made.

The emptiness I had lived with all my life was beginning to fill up with something so precious I can only venture to put a name on it. Spirituality is one, God is another, or maybe it was my soul, but those are all abstract concepts that can be argued ad infinitum with no increase in understanding. What is unarguable is the quality of the people who came into my life during this time.

There is a story about a skeptic who got lost in the wastes of Alaska. About to die from exposure, he prayed to a God he didn't believe in for help. Soon afterward an Eskimo came by and brought him back to civilization. Later the skeptic chided God, "Why didn't you help me when I was so desperately in need?" and God replied, "What do you want from me? I sent you an Eskimo, didn't I?" Rather than get involved in spiritual abstractions, I prefer to focus on tangibles—the Eskimos who turned up at this crucial point in my life to sustain, encourage, and love me when I was still unable to have kindly feelings toward myself.

One of my Eskimos is Terry Lamonde. I love the image of the crusty old mama she likes to portray. Her qualities of intensity and vivid individuality were what first struck me about her, but deeper than her style was a commitment to really *be* there for others. When I was with her I experienced what it was like to receive unconditional love, and it was so powerful I knew I was in contact with someone important, who had something to teach me about how to live life. I had no idea Terry was an Eskimo when I met her, but I have learned to identify them since as the people who come into your life when you are ready to learn something. She taught me to focus on what was really important, and to take risks in spite of my fears. She believed in me so strongly that I developed an equally strong desire to believe in myself.

Margaret was another Eskimo. She kept urging me to

go to college. "You help so many people," she said, "I really think you should become a psychologist." She even offered to baby-sit so I could go, and that impressed me. Marie, my sponsor, was another. She was not a bright woman, "just another alcoholic" to some, but to me she was special. She taught me how to give love and just be. She had an aura of simplicity about her that I really needed to understand. I felt like her daughter. There were many others, and their message was all the same: You can do it. I didn't believe in myself, but I believed in them.

I enrolled in the University of Central Florida shortly after I stopped drinking. I hadn't been in a classroom since the age of fifteen, half my life ago. I was still so obese I couldn't fit behind the desks, and my thoughts were so scattered I was afraid I had damaged my brain from alcohol. Full of fear, I was apologetic just for being there. I felt terribly isolated as I kept quiet and tried not to bother anybody. As awful as I felt, I went, day after day, until those feelings of inevitable failure began to dissipate and a few successes began to validate my right to be there.

Then I really took off. Always an extremist, I became supercharged. Working part-time as a waitress and carrying as many as twenty-four hours a semester, I managed to earn a four-year degree in psychology in less than three years. Not even a bout with cancer of the cervix was able to slow me down. Instead of congratulating me on my degree, Marie urged me to go on and get a master's. By this time, I had come to believe that I could do anything, and I went on to get an advanced degree. I wanted it for myself, but I also wanted it for Marie, who was dying of cancer. Toward the end, when she was too ill to go out, I brought about ten people to her house and we had a meeting. The topic was acceptance. She sat in a chair and talked about her fear of dying alone, and there was so much love in her I knew she couldn't really die. The feelings we all had for her wouldn't stop when her body ceased to function.

I brought her to the hospital the following Monday. Four days later I woke up knowing Marie was waiting for me to come to her so she could die, and I avoided going to see her. Suddenly, walking aimlessly around a shopping mall, I said to myself, What are you doing here? and ran to my car. When I walked into her hospital room, she was in a coma, but I knew she knew I was there. I told her, "I'm here with you," and held her and talked to her until she died in my arms. Marie's legacy to me was to go out and be an Eskimo, to give to others what she had given to me: her simplicity and her unconditional love. She lives through me.

While getting my master's degree, I worked part-time in the Navy's alcohol rehab program, a joint venture with the University of West Florida. With my usual zeal, I became first a facilitator, then a screener, next a coordinator, and finally a trainer of facilitators. Because I was addicted to food as well as alcohol, I wanted the center to treat both, and tried to convince the director, to begin to look at food as an addictive substance. He was reluctant at first, having worked hard just to get alcoholism recognized as a disease, and was concerned that bringing in food addiction would dilute the program. I understood his reluctance. No treatment centers were treating food addictions at the time, and the Navy is not known to be an institution that encourages maverick thinking. Compliance is what they value. But I had been a maverick all my life and I persisted. I felt like a pioneer. I was a pioneer.

I believe you can educate someone who abuses a substance into recovery but not an addict. I had been educated plenty—by my humiliation in the airplane that couldn't take off, by the horrors of finding ways to eat after having my mouth wired, and by a thousand other painful lessons—and so I knew no amount of education got me to stop behaving addictively. I argued that treatment had to go beyond detoxifying the body and educating the mind. Addiction is also a disease of the emotions, and no amount of intellectual understanding will treat them in any meaningful way. My logic was, instead of focusing on the substance, the external disease, we should focus on the whole person—the body, mind, emotions, and spirit—helping people break through their defensive self-destructive behavior patterns to get them to change what they were doing in their life *today*, to give them tools that would allow them to create an identity for themselves and set them free.

My persistence paid off. I opened up an alcohol rehab center that was therapeutic and 12-step oriented. Unlike other treatment centers I had heard about where people were shamed and humiliated, I stressed love, acceptance, safety—all the things I had discovered I needed in order to change. It worked. People did change. Like me, they dared to take risks and turn their lives around. The program was so successful it became a model for other treatment centers.

When I first came into the fellowship, I was taught that fear and faith can't live in the same house. I bought that idea, and I used to worry when I was afraid that I was doing something wrong. Now I believe I will probably always have fear in my life. When I speak from a podium in front of thousands of people, I'm absolutely petrified. Sometimes I'm afraid just to get up in front of a group of patients. I'm not as articulate as I would like to be, and sometimes I beat myself up about that.

I've learned to think of fear as part of my nature and have made the choice either to act with fear, or fear and take no action. Over the years, I've always chosen the action. I tell myself fear is just another feeling and act in spite of the way I feel, and that is what has made me successful. When people protest by saying it doesn't feel good to be afraid, I say, it doesn't matter. Acknowledge the fear and do what you know is right in your heart. Good things will come from that.

When I opened the first center in 1986, my heart was pounding. Most people are advised not to launch a new business unless they've got the security of a substantial amount of capital to float on. My capital was more the size of a rowboat than a cruise ship, and that made me full of fear. I was told by the bank that I might get the money I needed to start operating the center in a few months, but I couldn't wait that long and borrowed $100,000 on my own. A friend of mine had received $50,000 that had been willed to her, and her grateful husband added another $50,000 to that. Then I went out and got every kind of credit card I could get my hands on, over twenty of them, and that's how I financed the center. Most people won't do that because they need to feel secure. I took my insecurity and did it anyway.

Buddy also played an important part in motivating me to start the center. We were born on the same day, and when he came into the program at five hundred pounds, I became his close friend. I was also close to his wife and daughter. Buddy was an artist and did beautiful graphics and artwork for a conference we worked on together. Just before the conference, he died. He was one of numerous people in the program we had lost from their addiction that year, and I was angry that we had all these treatment centers for alcoholism but there wasn't any really structured help for food addiction. I took that anger and used it as energy to motivate myself to make a difference, to deal with something that had always been neglected by society, and to help other people like my beloved Buddy live long, full, and useful lives.

In opening up the centers my motivation has never been to make money. I use the same approach to financial success that I do with food addiction: In order to conquer the latter you do not try to conquer it, and in order to be a financial success, you do not try to make money. I have made a lot of money and I spend it just as fast. Money is not a priority. God, family, and friends are my priority. Good begets good that comes back to me as more good—it's contagious!

There's a saying that I have adopted as one of my guides through life: "Die young—as late as possible." Youthfulness to me means the ability to take active participation in creating one's own destiny, to be willing to risk failure and rejection, and to be resilient when the failure and rejection inevitably occur. The incredible life force within us is available to anyone who wishes to tap into it. But it often becomes blocked by depression, which inhibits our ability to be absorbed in what's happening in the present and causes us to dwell on the past.

Boredom is an early indication of a slip back into depression, and at 42 percent, the most frequent cause of relapse—more than social situations or emotional issues!

Boredom is about not really living life. It's about falling into a passive form of existence, a desire to be entertained rather than to actively entertain life's great and often unexpected possibilities. Sometimes people in early recovery slip into the habit of watching too much television, which only increases their boredom. Next thing you know, they start succumbing to all those tantalizing food commercials and decide to eat to relieve their boredom. Unless they pull themselves out of their lethargy into purposeful activity, they can fall right back into the addictive cycle.

People who make a contribution and have a purpose in life are never bored. There's so much to do! When I was on the sidelines of life, controlled by my addiction, I didn't know what my purpose was, or have a clue as to the kind of contributions I could make. Today, there are not enough hours in the day to do everything I want to do. Since 1986, the number of my treatment centers has increased seven-fold and we're still growing. I have also formed an agency that specializes in insurance and financial planning for women. I am excited about publishing a magazine called "For Us" and my clothing line, Janet Greeson's For Us by David Dow, offers the glamour, fun and expression that is rarely available in "great" women's sizes.

Yet, I swear to you, there's nothing unique or special about me. If I can do it, you can do it. God gives all of us gifts. Some put gifts in a closet, but I relish the gifts I get, use them to maximize my contribution to life and have received so much real nourishment in return.

I am a model of recovery. Today I really believe I'm God's kid and that has made all the difference.

The loneliness I have carried around with me all my life is still with me at times, but most of the time I really feel as if my cup runneth over. I possess an energy I know is more than the sum of my parts, which I don't try to analyze. I know people who are married or in a relationship who experience a more severe kind of emptiness than I do. When that void begins to ache, I see the little girl within me who didn't understand and I embrace her. There is only one person in the world who can help her, and that's God and me. When I am nurturing her, I am not angry or filled with fear. I feel good about being able to take care of myself, I don't have to give my all to a man, and I feel good about that, too. For some reason men find that intriguing. Maybe they realize there's a part of me they're never going to get. They sense the power of my boundaries and that attracts them.

My mother and I have a unique relationship in that she's my best friend and I enjoy being with her. I'm aware how rare that is between mothers and daughters and am grateful for it. We live in proximity but maintain our private lives. We work together and help each other solve our daily problems and know that no matter what happens we will be there for each other. We've grown beyond mother-daughter to mainstays.

My deepest and strongest relationships are with my three children. They each give me something special. Gene, my oldest, gives me his 100 percent acceptance. He loves and understands me, and I him. When he was in high school, he always scored low on intelligence and aptitude tests, and his high school counselors laughed at him when he said he wanted to go to college. I told him, "Gene, you can do anything. You're going to college." I drilled into him that his test scores didn't matter, and I told him my story about how intelligence is like a glass of water: People can have half a glass, a quarter of a glass, or a full glass. It doesn't matter how intelligent they are, it's what they do with what they have.

Gene went to college, first to Loyola, then Notre Dame, and he graduated from Tulane. He's very successful today with a career in the Navy.

Jimmy is a lover and an old soul. He looks mischievous with his long hair and dancing eyes, a second-generation hippie. His face reveals his wisdom, that he knows what's really important. He's a musician who plays electric guitar and he's going to be famous one day. I know that he will always be there for me, no matter what, and I for him.

Rosemary lights up my life. She radiates joyfulness. If I spend just a few minutes in her presence, she energizes me, and I see that happen with others just as much as with me. She inspires people and also accepts them, just as they are. Her message is simple but clear—she wants them to be happy. All three of my kids are a strong part of the ebb and flow of my life. I give to them, but they also give back to me, and I think that's important. I get the impression from a lot of parents that we should just give and give to our kids and not expect anything back, but that's stressful, and I see this one-sidedness particularly in addictive families. I believe the flow of love has to go both ways so that everyone is constantly replenished.

I have learned to live in the middle spectrum of emotions, where addicts are so uncomfortable, because I find that there I can remain on a more even keel. That way the intensity isn't there when I make mistakes, either. Other people are often devastated when things go wrong, but I'm usually not. For instance, in alcoholism treatment I believe that I don't get them drunk and I don't get them sober. When there are accolades about the treatment and people pay compliments, I don't pick them up. The other side is, when something goes wrong, I don't pick that up, either. I just don't need external validation because I get that from within.

I save my excitement for recovery. I know I'm God's kid and that gives me a zest for living. I know He has better plans for me than I could ever dream up. I know that I'm a messenger, an Eskimo, and that my spirituality doesn't belong to me but works through me. I just keep showing up and do what I believe I've been put on this earth to do. In my over fifteen years of recovery, I've come to believe in the saying that it's not the end of the journey that matters, it's the journey that matters in the end. I travel light. I enjoy the trip. I'm still excited about recovery. I'm real, and that's all that matters.

JANET GREESON, Ph.D.

Workbook for Chapter Five

Write your autobiography, beginning with your earliest memory. Emphasize emotions, not facts. Include significant people and events that made you what you are today. Write down the messages about yourself you received from these significant people, and the memories of food connected with feelings that go back to your childhood. Be sure to include secrets you kept, and benchmarks, those revelatory moments when you got a new perspective on your life up to that point. Include the history of addiction in your family on both sides where appropriate, the onset of your addictive behavior, and the progression of your addiction.

At this point, you may not feel you have much to write about recovery, but you have just finished a book that has powerfully affected your capacity for change, provided you have done the necessary work. Reflect on changes you have already made, and how the positive feedback from those changes has encouraged you to continue.

This autobiography is meant to be open-ended. In the weeks and months to come, it will have new meaning for you, and you will want to add to the recovery section. Keep it always. It is a legacy of your courage, and it will increase in value to you as the years go by.

Affirmation for the Rest of My Life

I am not my body
I am free
I am as God created me
I am part of a community
I am safe and strong
In my own company
For I am not my body
I am free.

THE TWELVE STEPS OF ALCOHOLICS ANONYMOUS

1. We admitted we were powerless over alcohol—that our lives had become unmanageable.
2. Came to believe that a Power greater than ourselves could restore us to sanity.
3. Made a decision to turn our will and our lives over to the care of God *as we understood him*.
4. Made a searching and fearless moral inventory of ourselves.
5. Admitted to God, to ourselves, and to another human being the exact nature of our wrongs.
6. Were entirely ready to have God remove all these defects of character.
7. Humbly asked Him to remove our shortcomings.
8. Made a list of all persons we had harmed, and became willing to make amends to them all.
9. Made direct amends to such people wherever possible, except when to do so would injure them or others.
10. Continued to take personal inventory and when we were wrong promptly admitted it.
11. Sought through prayer and meditation to improve our conscious contact with God *as we understood Him,* praying only for knowledge of His will for us and the power to carry that out.
12. Having had a spiritual awakening as the result of these Steps, we tried to carry this message to alcoholics, and to practice these principles in all our affairs.
